A Taste of English

A Nutrition Workbook for Adult ESL Students

Student Workbook

Acknowledgements

Special thanks to:

Donald Sykes
Director
Office of Community Services

Maiso Bryant
Branch Chief
Office of Financial Management
Division of Discretionary Grants

Joseph Carrol
Program Manager
OCS

Joseph Reid
Acting Division Director
Discretionary Grants, OCS

Lorraine Berry
Grants Specialist
OFM/DDG

ESL Nutrition Advisory Workgroup:

Patricia Bernstein
Faculty Assistant
Maryland Cooperative
Extension Office

Gerardo Martinez
Project Director
University Research Corporation/
Center for Human Services

Patty Symonette
Embassy of the Bahamas

Darby Eliades
Senior Project Associate
National Center for Education
in Maternal and Child Health

Ada Mejia
ESL Housing Service Administrator
Rural Opportunities Inc.

Myrna Tarrant
ESL Specialist and Nutritionist
Fairfax County Adult and
Community Education Program

Susan Joyner
Adult Education Staff
Development Specialist
Virginia Commonwealth University

Sandra Mottola
WIC Nutritionist
Arlington County
Department of Human Services

Tony Traywick
ESL Coordinator
Telamon Corporation

Fran Keenan
Assistant Director for
National Clearinghouse for ESL Literacy Education
Center for Applied Linguistics

Pretesters: Diana De Bor, Fred Johnson, Sue Mathison, Suzanne Pate, and Cruz Rodriguez. We also thank the numerous field-testers for their assistance in ensuring that this publication is user-friendly.

ISBN 1-886567-04-2

© 1994. Additional Copies of *A Taste of English* are available from AFOP. Portions may be reproduced with permission.

Table of Contents

Lesson 1: Be Good to Your Body 1

Lesson 2: Know How Your Body Works 21

Lesson 3: Eat a Variety of Foods 31

Lesson 4: Make Healthy Meals 47

Lesson 5: Keep Foods Safe 63

Lesson 6: Be a Smart Shopper 79

Lesson 7: Eat Well and Stay Healthy 95

Lesson 8: Get the Help You Need 107

Glossary of Foods 123

1 2 3 4 5 6 7 8

Be Good to Your Body

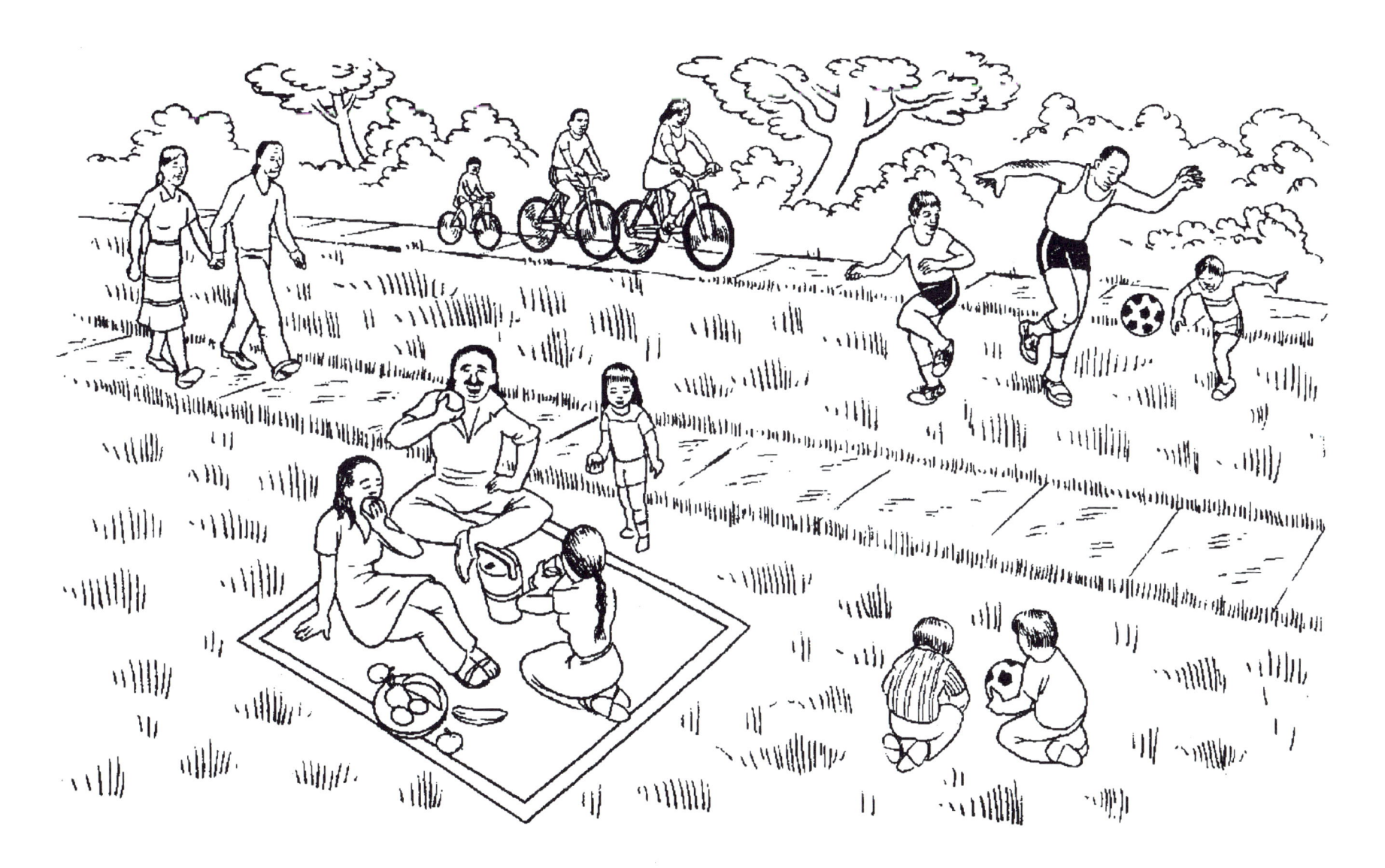

1. Eat healthy foods.

bread, cereal, rice, and pasta

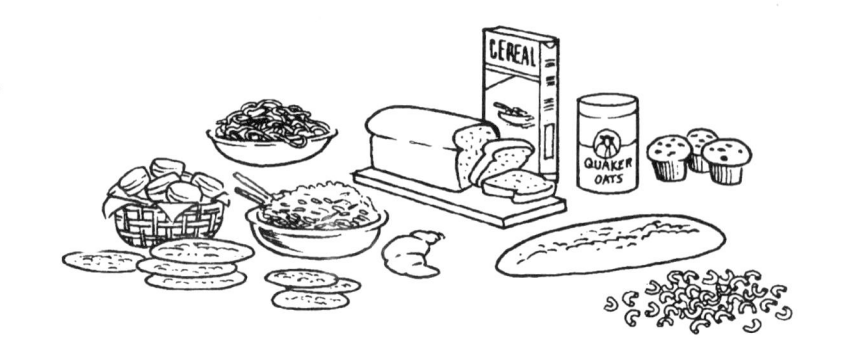

vegetables

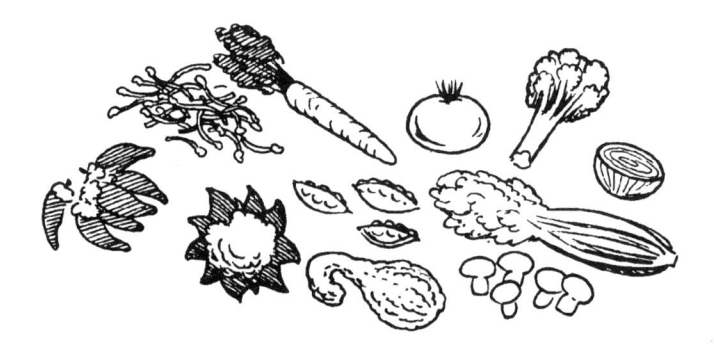

fruit

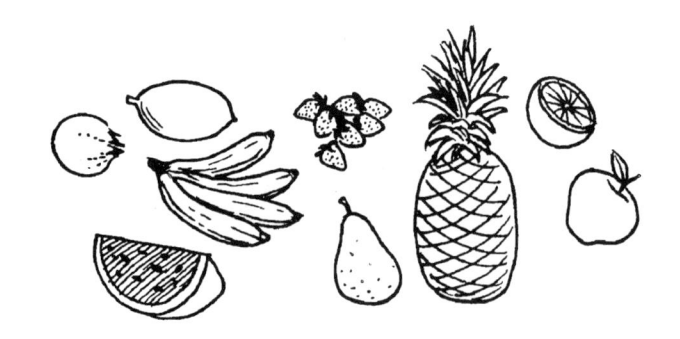

meat, poultry, fish, beans, eggs, and nuts

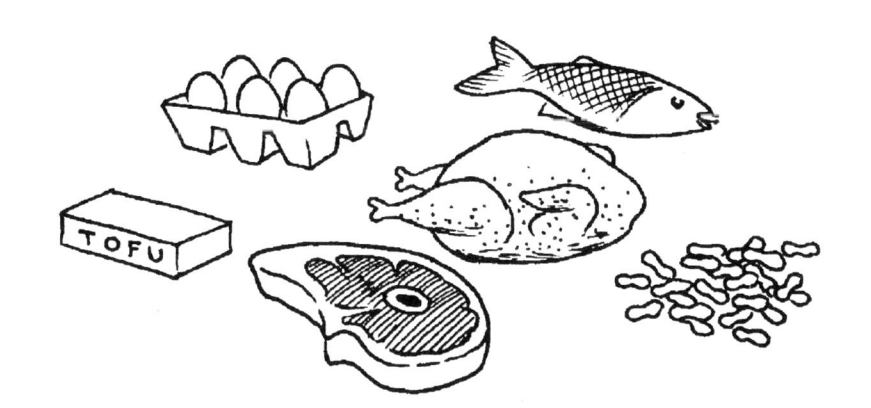

milk, yogurt, and cheese

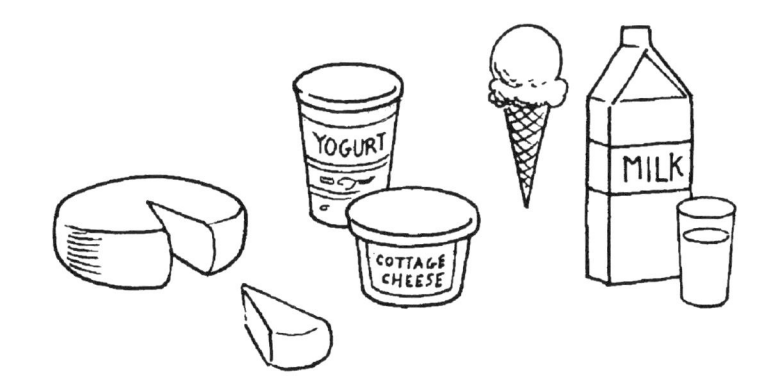

Lesson 1

2. Watch your weight.

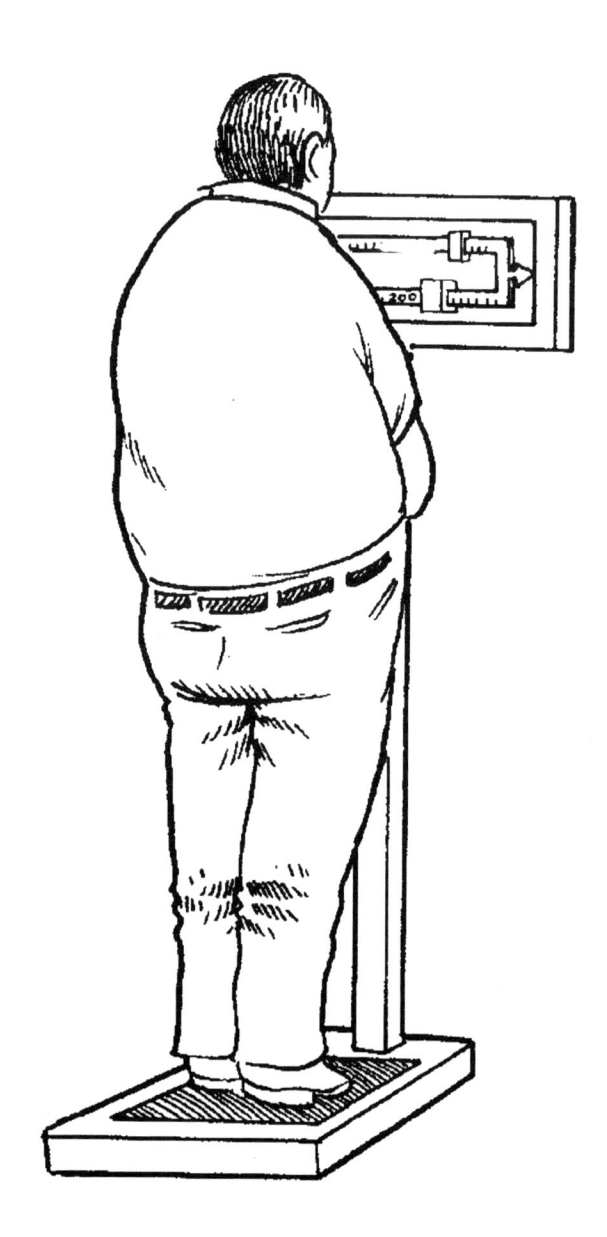

Find your weight.

Weights for Adults

Height	Weight in pounds	
	19 to 34 years	35 years and over
5'0"	97-128	108-138
5'1"	101-132	111-143
5'2"	104-137	115-148
5'3"	107-141	119-152
5'4"	111-146	122-157
5'5"	114-150	126-162
5'6"	118-155	130-167
5'7"	121-160	134-172
5'8"	125-164	138-178
5'9"	129-169	142-183
5'10"	132-174	146-188
5'11"	136-179	151-194
6'0"	140-184	155-199
6'1"	144-189	159-205

Source: Derived from the National Research Council, 1989.

Lesson 1

Calories are energy.

Too many calories and no exercise can make you overweight.

Few Calories

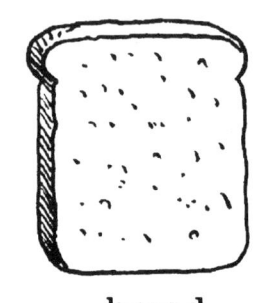

bread
60 calories per slice

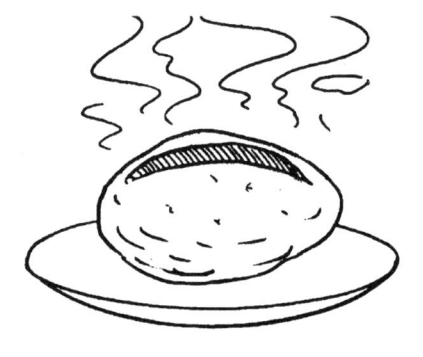

potato
100 calories

Many Calories

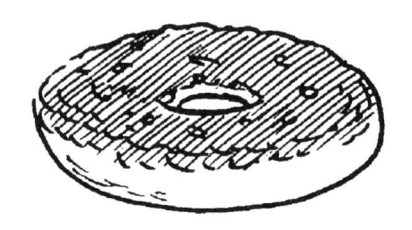

donut
245 calories

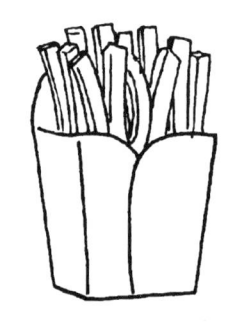

french fries
320 calories

Few Calories

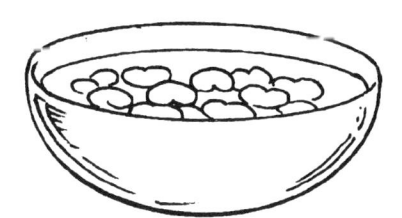

beans
60 calories

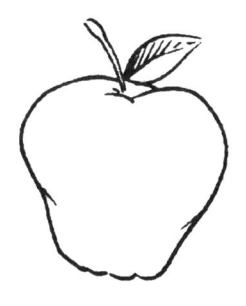

apple
80 calories

Many Calories

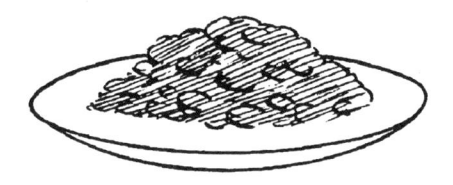

refried beans
150 calories

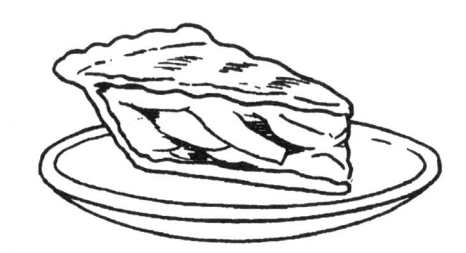

apple pie
405 calories

Lesson 1

Which food has more calories? Circle it.

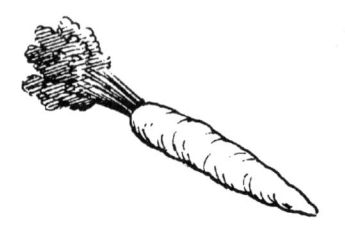

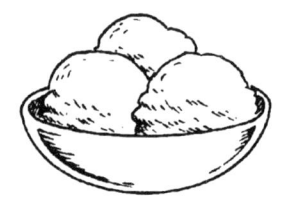

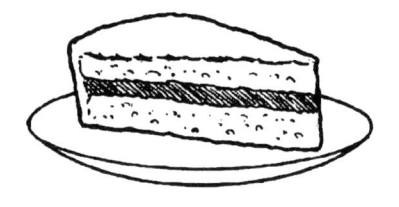

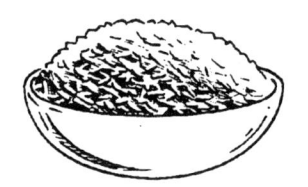

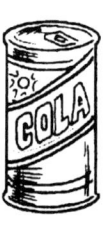

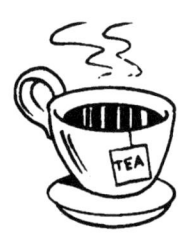

1. carrot / ice cream

2. cake / rice

3. soda / tea

3. Eat less fat.

Too much fat in your diet can hurt you.

Low Fat

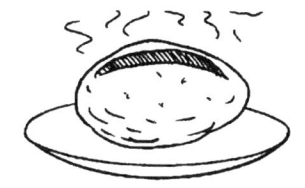

potato
0 grams of fat

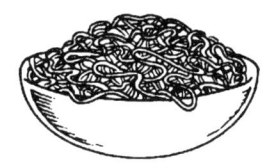

noodles
2 grams of fat

High Fat

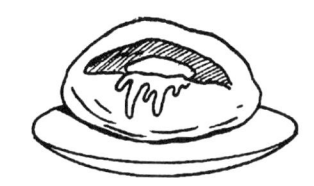

potato with butter
4 grams of fat

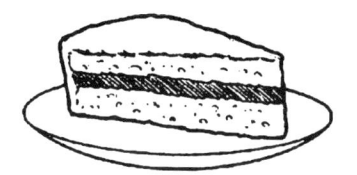

cake
17 grams of fat

How much fat can you eat?

Daily Calories	Who?	Daily Fat Grams (30% of calories)
1600	Women	60-80 grams of fat
2200	Men	75-105 grams of fat

Lesson 1

What other foods are high in fat?

1. _____ 2. _____

3. _____ 4. _____

What foods do you eat?

1. _____ 2. _____

3. _____ 4. _____

Are these foods high fat or low fat?

4. Drink more water.

Water is very important for the body.

Drink eight glasses of water a day.

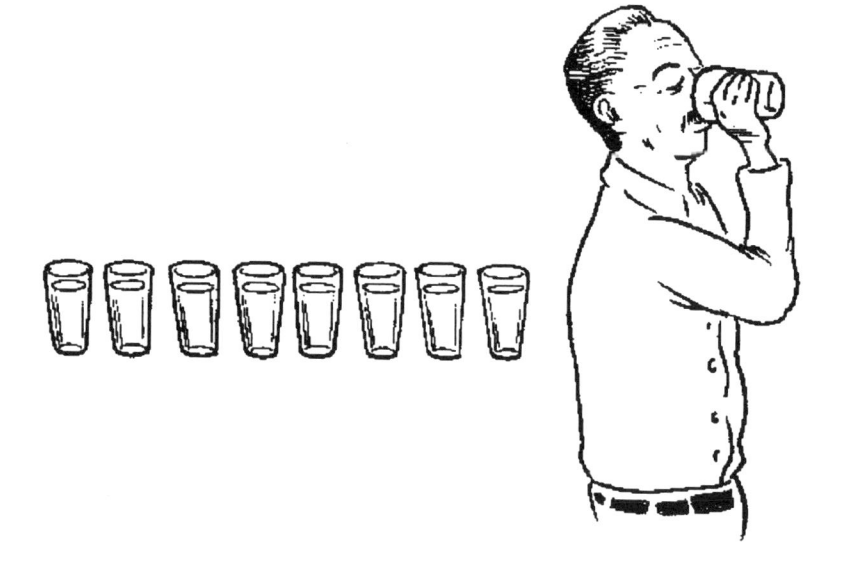

5. Eat more fiber.

Fiber is important for digestion.

Fiber is in vegetables, fruits, beans and grains.

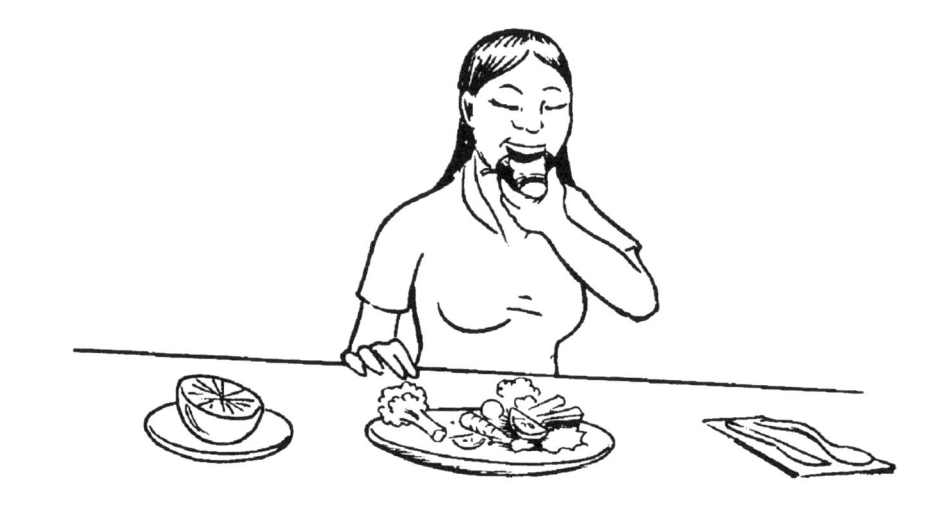

6. Don't smoke.

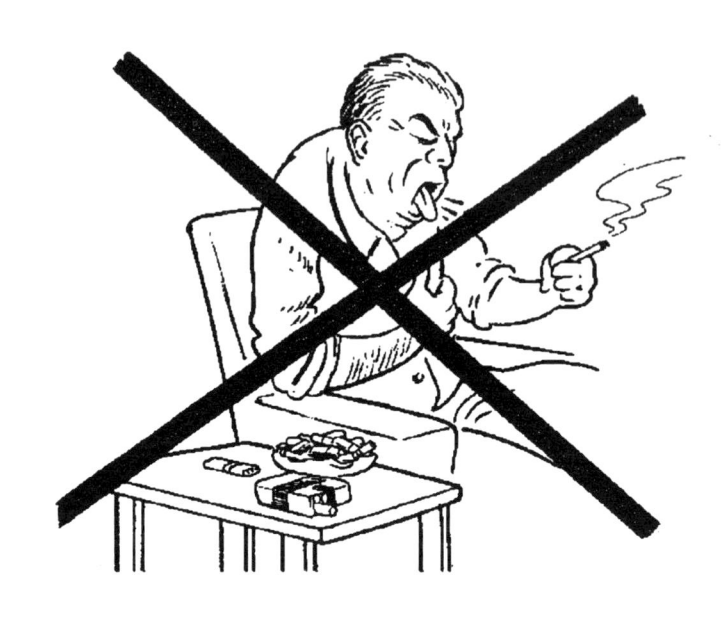

7. Have less caffeine.

Caffeine can make you nervous.

It is in coffee, tea, some sodas,

and chocolate.

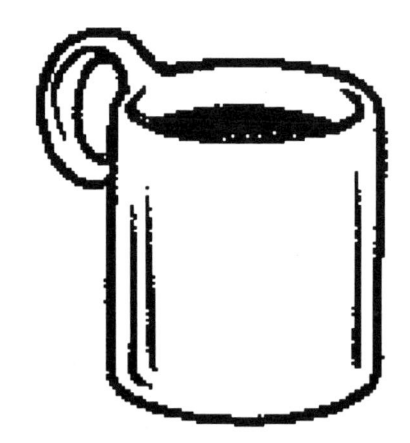

8. Drink less alcohol.

Alcohol is in beer, wine,

and other liquor.

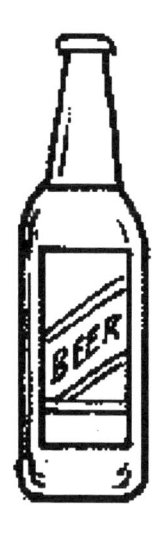

9. Eat less salt and sodium.

Salt has sodium. Some packaged foods have sodium.

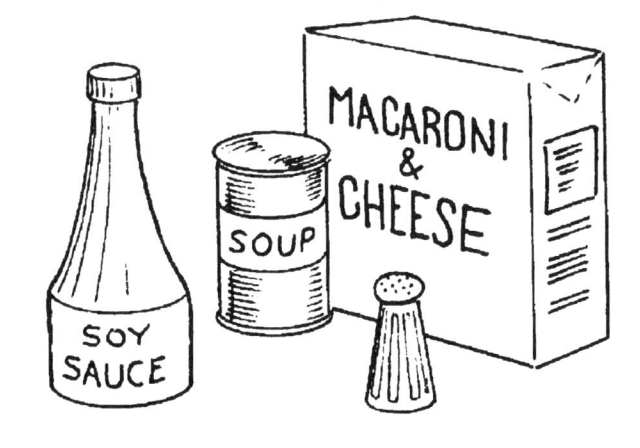

Lesson 1

10. Exercise more.

Exercise makes your heart and muscles strong. It burns calories. Exercise 3 times a week for 20 minutes. Ask your doctor first.

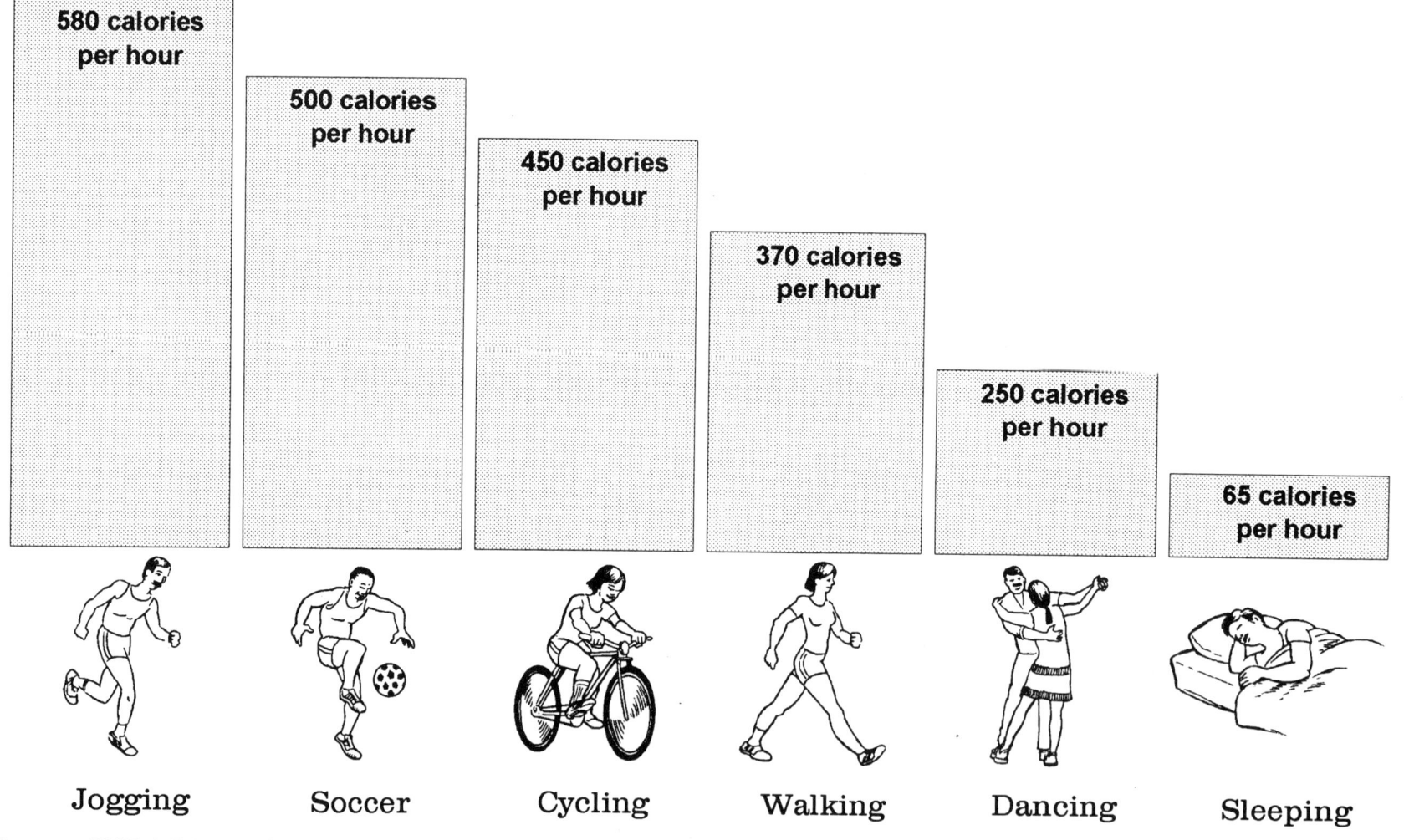

Jogging	580 calories per hour
Soccer	500 calories per hour
Cycling	450 calories per hour
Walking	370 calories per hour
Dancing	250 calories per hour
Sleeping	65 calories per hour

Source: USDA Dietary Guidelines, 7/93.

Do you exercise?

When?	What?	How Long?
Sunday	walk	20 minutes
Sunday		
Monday		
Tuesday		
Wednesday		
Thursday		
Friday		
Saturday		

Lesson 1

Match the pictures with the words.

a. Don't smoke.

b. Watch your weight.

c. Eat less sodium.

d. Exercise more.

e. Drink less alcohol.

f. Eat healthy foods.

g. Eat more fiber.

h. Use less caffeine.

i. Eat less fat.

j. Drink more water.

Look at the pictures and the words. Match the pictures with the words. Write the correct letter in the boxes below.

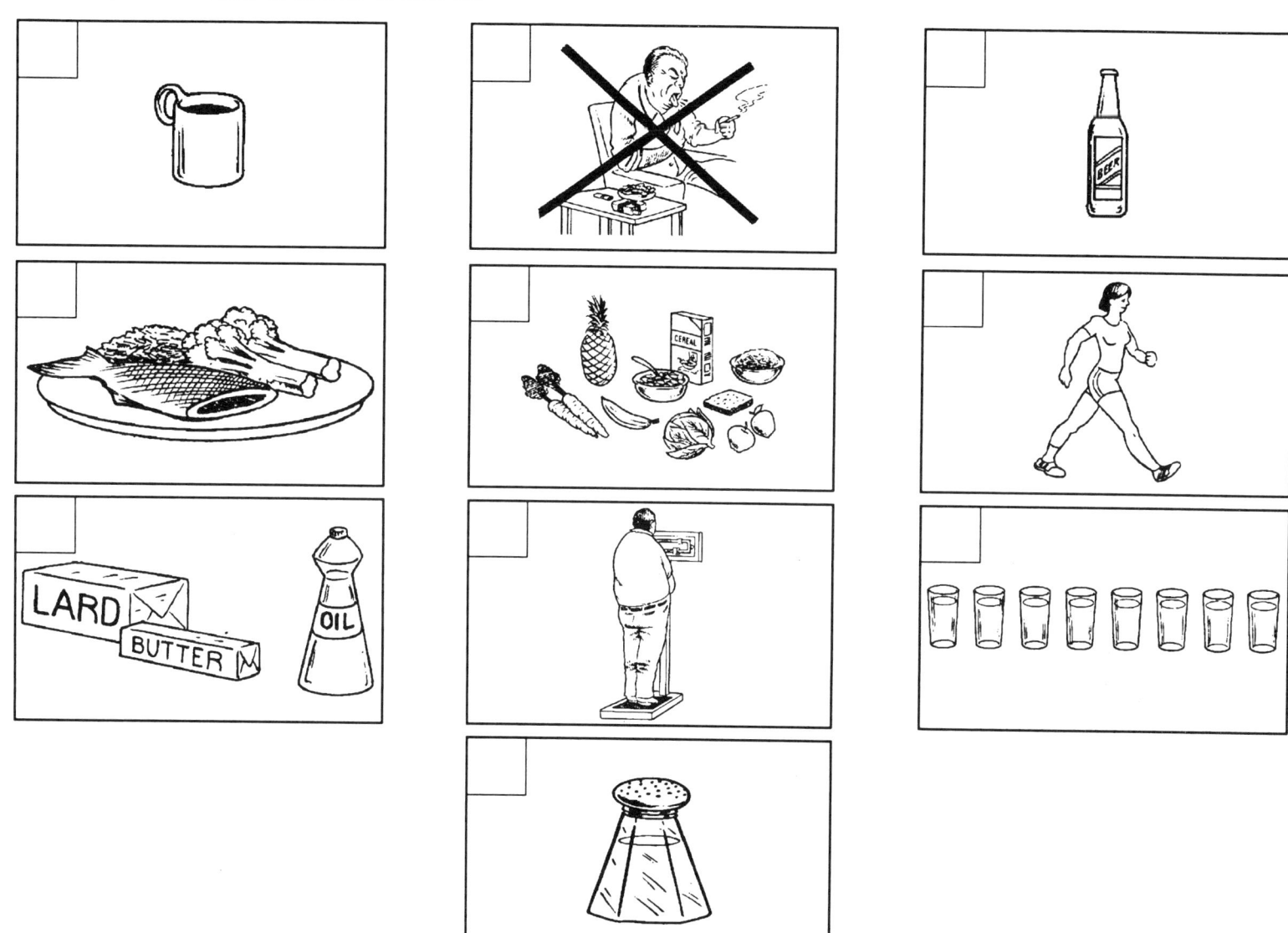

Fred

Fred wants a healthy body. Tell him what to do.

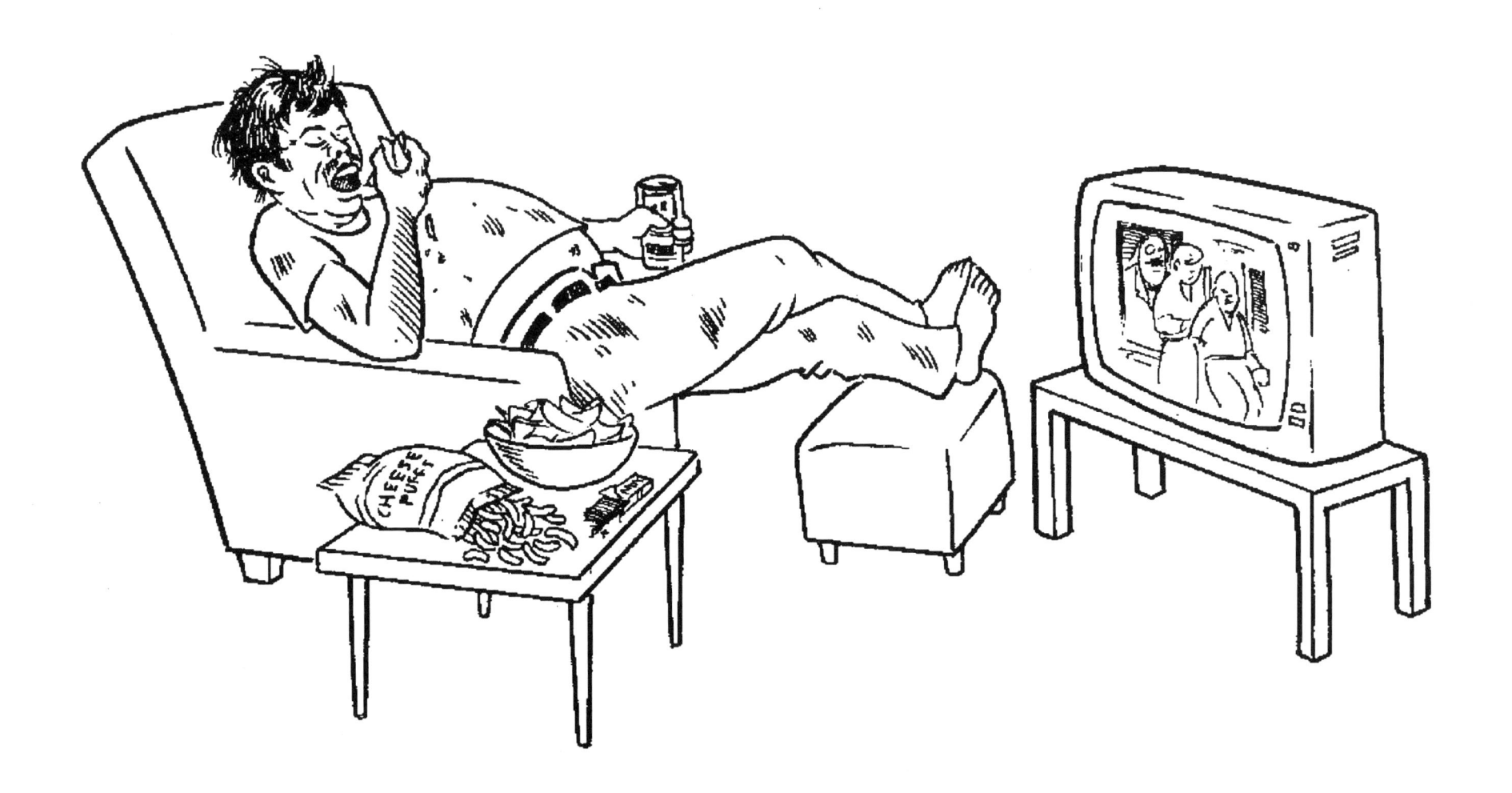

Write the answers.

1. Eat _____ foods.

2. _____ _____ weight.

3. Eat less _____.

4. Drink more _____.

5. Eat more _____.

6. Use less _____.

7. Drink less _____.

8. Eat less _____.

9. Don't _____.

10. _____ _____.

What other things can you tell Fred?

Lesson 1

A Healthy Recipe

Fruit Salad

3 peaches
1/4 cantaloupe
2 apples

1/2 cup blueberries
3 tablespoons cherries
1 cup strawberries

1. Wash the peaches. Remove the peel. Dice into bite-size pieces. Put pieces in a bowl.

2. Cut the rind off the cantaloupe. Dice the slices into bite-size pieces. Put the pieces in the bowl.

3. Wash the apples and core them. Then dice them into bite-size pieces. Place in bowl.

4. Wash the blueberries. Add them to the other fruits.

5. Wash the strawberries. Pull off the green tops. Slice each strawberry. Add to bowl.

6. Wash cherries. Take the pits out of them. Add to other fruits.

7. Mix all fruits together. Place in dishes. *Makes 6 servings.*

1 **2** 3 4 5 6 7 8

Know How Your Body Works

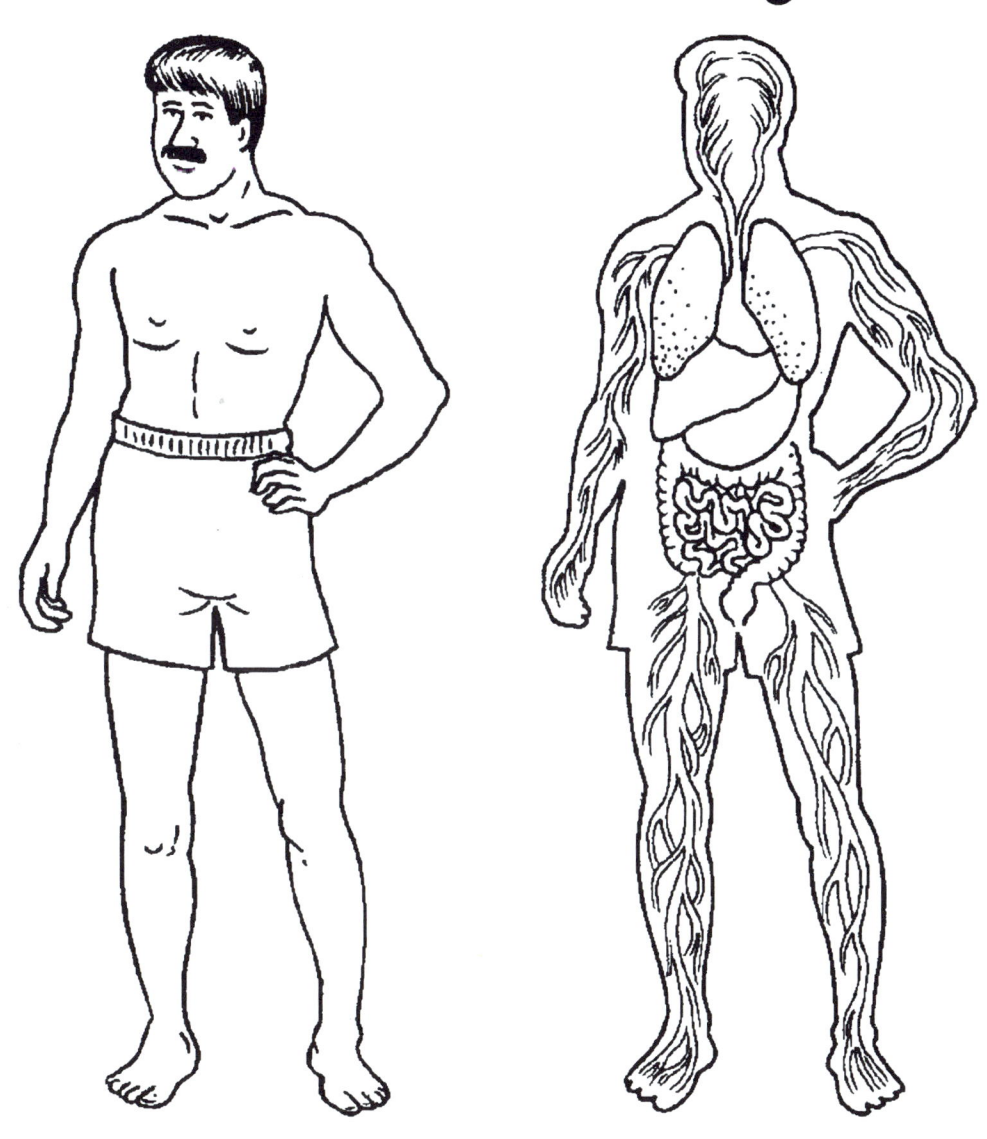

Lesson 2

Your Body

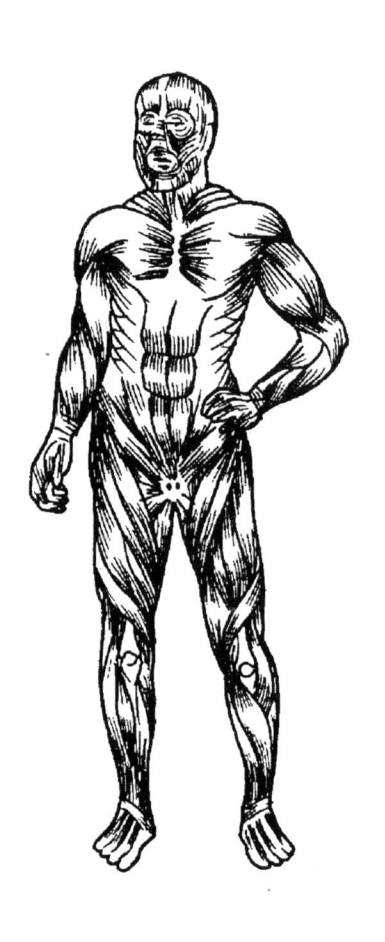

Muscles make your body move.

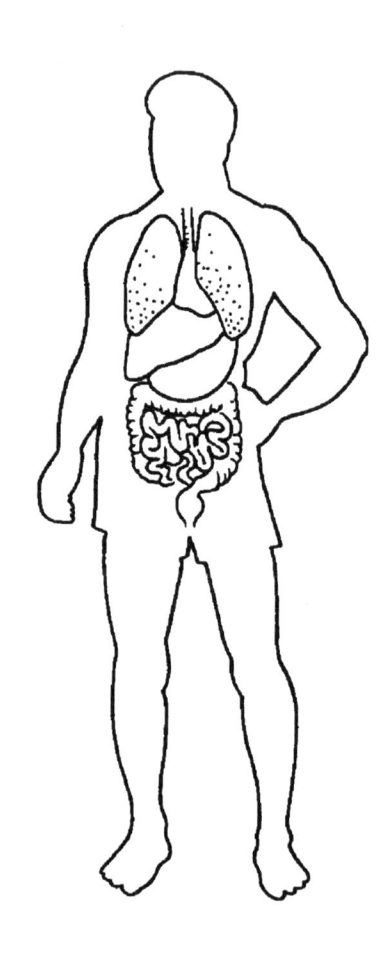

Organs work to make us live.

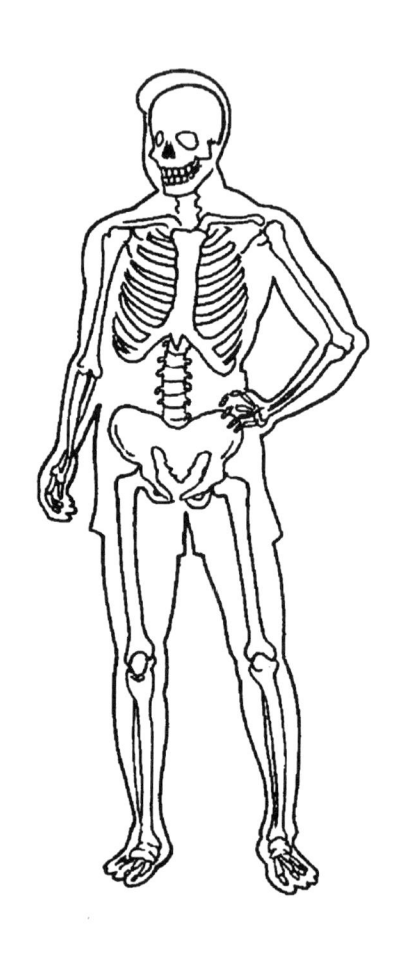

Bones help your body stand straight.

Circulation

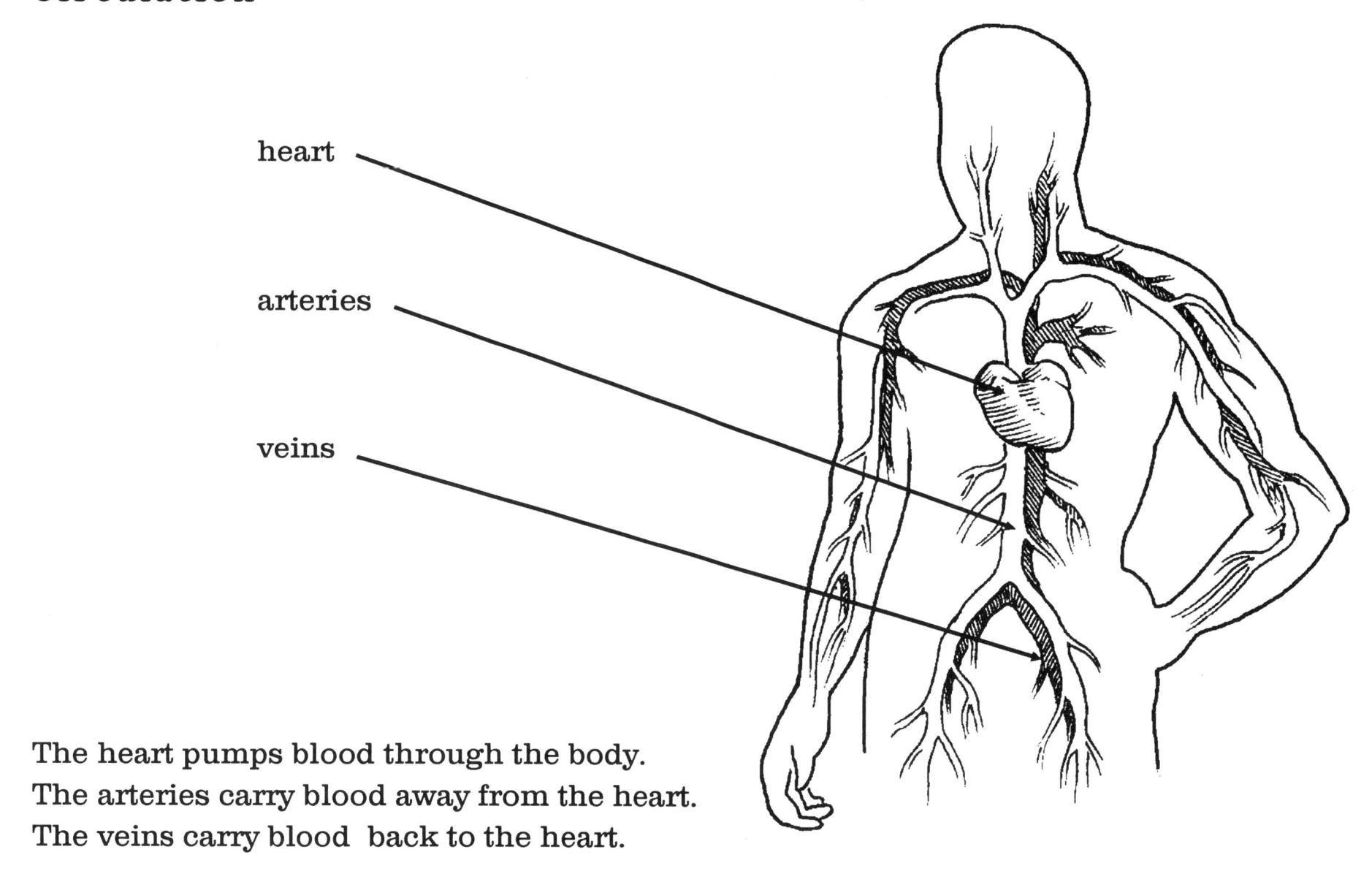

heart

arteries

veins

The heart pumps blood through the body.
The arteries carry blood away from the heart.
The veins carry blood back to the heart.

Eat well and exercise to keep your heart healthy.

Your body makes cholesterol from the fat you eat. Cholesterol can make your arteries narrow. The heart must work hard to pump blood through small arteries.

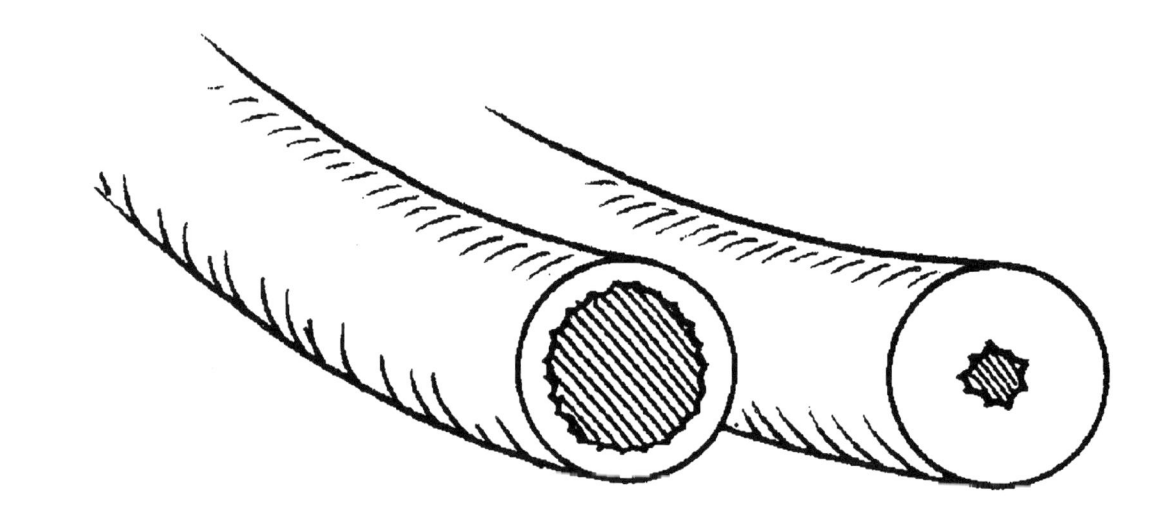

You can help your heart.

Sodium is in salt and some other foods. Too much sodium can make your blood pressure high. High blood pressure can make you sick.

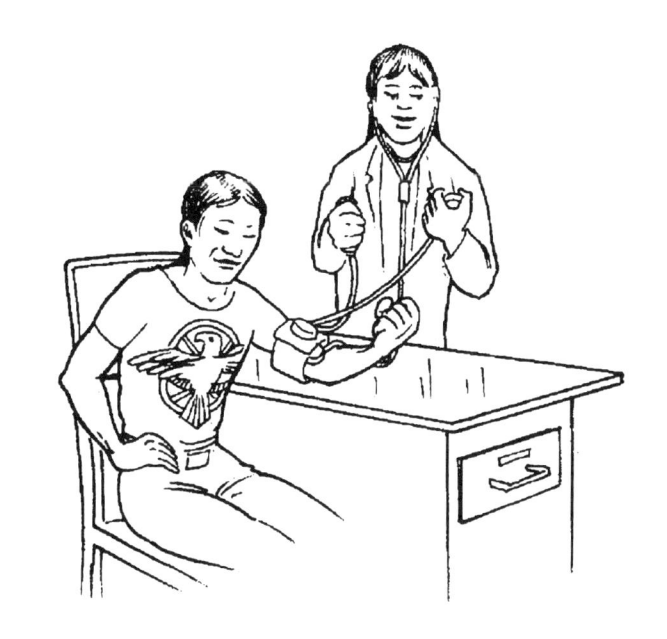

Caffeine can make you nervous. There is caffeine in coffee, tea, some sodas, and chocolate. How many cups of coffee do you drink every day?

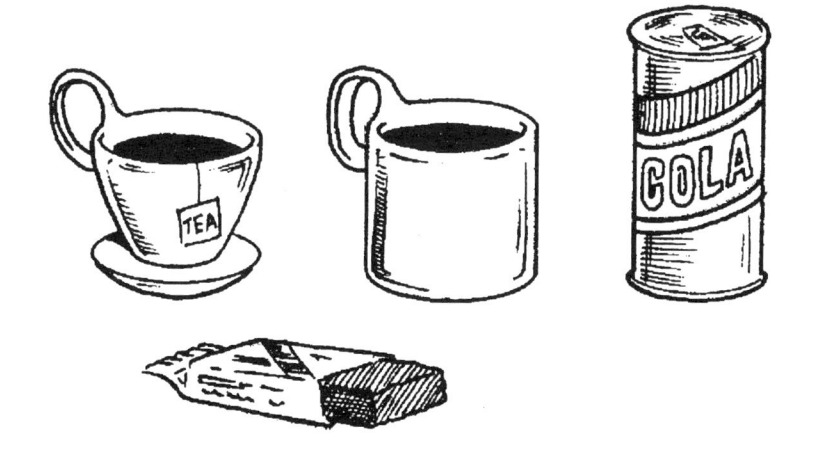

_____

Digestion

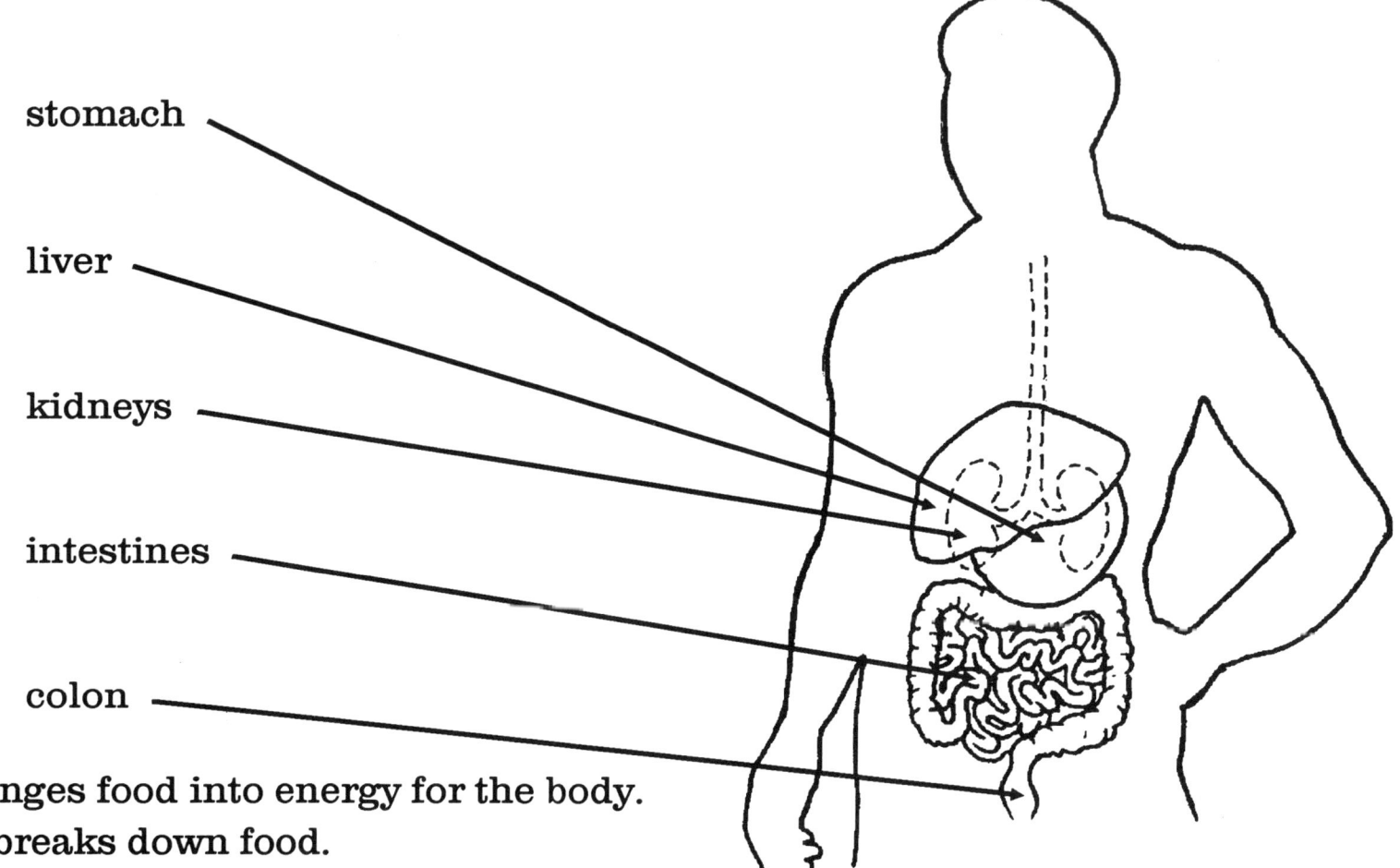

stomach

liver

kidneys

intestines

colon

Digestion changes food into energy for the body.
The stomach breaks down food.
The liver removes poisons from food.
The kidneys remove water from food.
The intestines take in food the body can use. The intestines also change the food the body cannot use into waste.
The colon passes the waste out of the body.

You can help digestion.

Drink more water.

Eat more fiber.

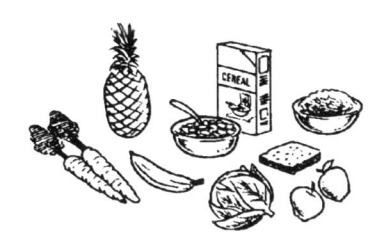

Too much alcohol is bad for the liver.

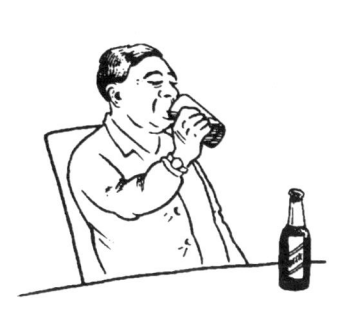

Circle True (T) or False (F).

1. The intestines remove poisons from the food.   T   F
2. The colon passes the waste out of the body.   T   F
3. The kidneys break down food.   T   F
4. The stomach removes water from the food.   T   F
5. The liver takes in food the body can use.   T   F
6. The intestines also change the food the body cannot use into waste.   T   F

Lesson 2

Respiration

Your lungs breathe air in and out of your body.

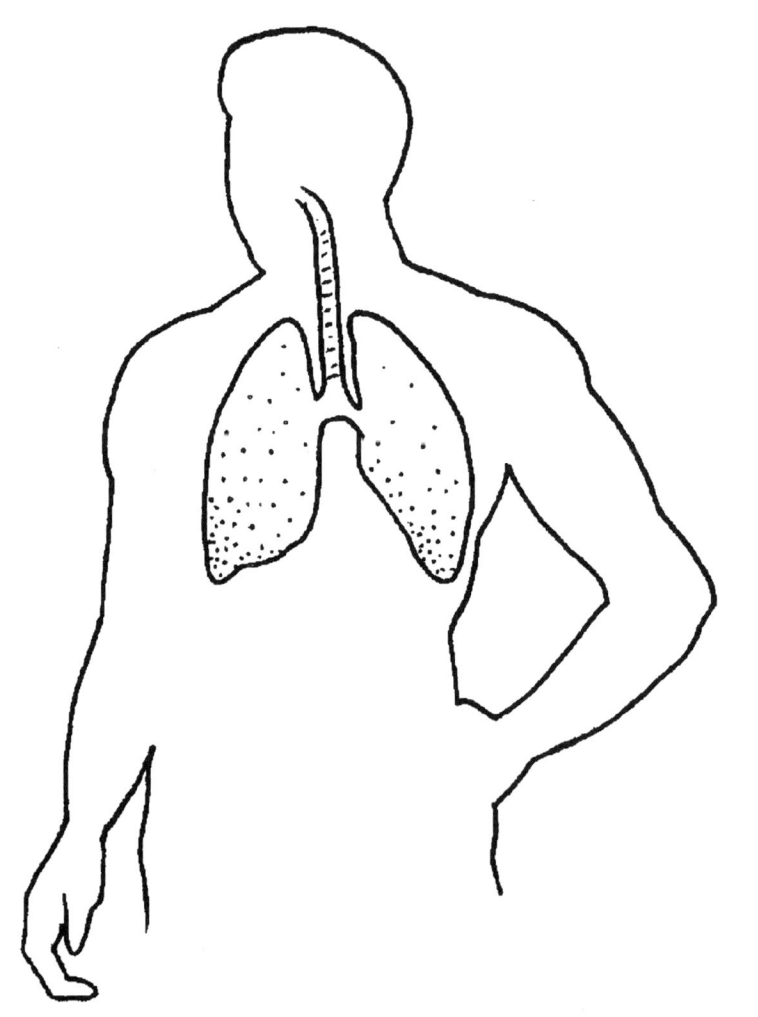

Don't smoke! It's bad for the lungs.

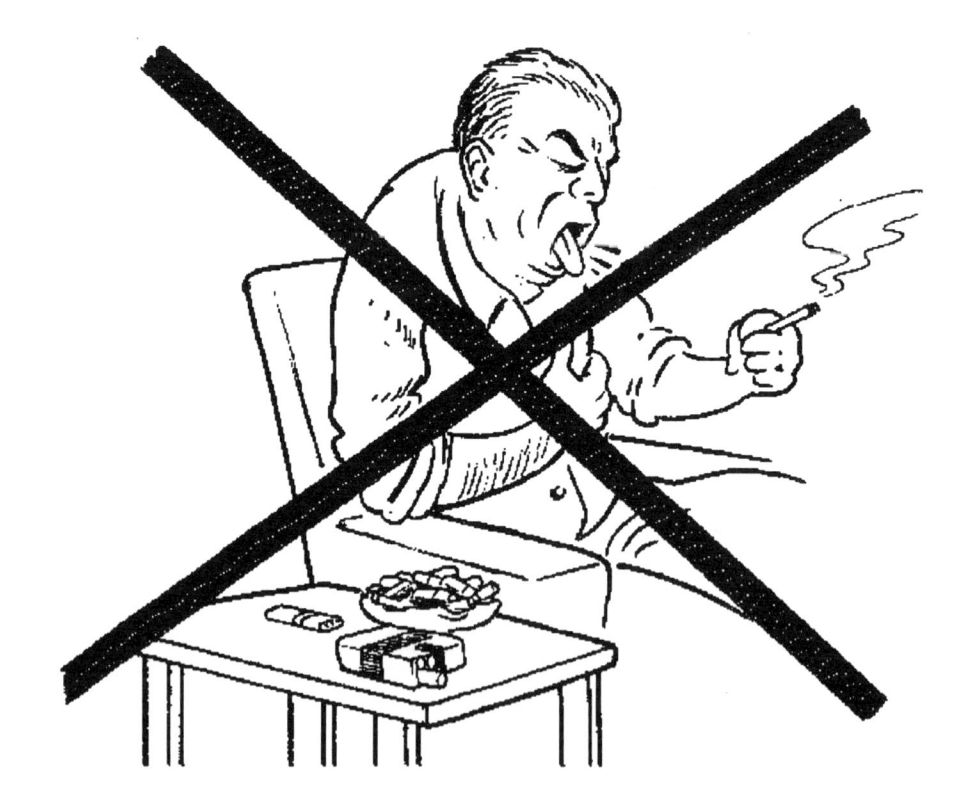

The Body

Fill in the blanks.

1. _____
2. _____
3. _____
4. _____
5. _____
6. _____
7. _____
8. _____

heart   stomach   lungs

arteries   liver   colon

veins   intestines

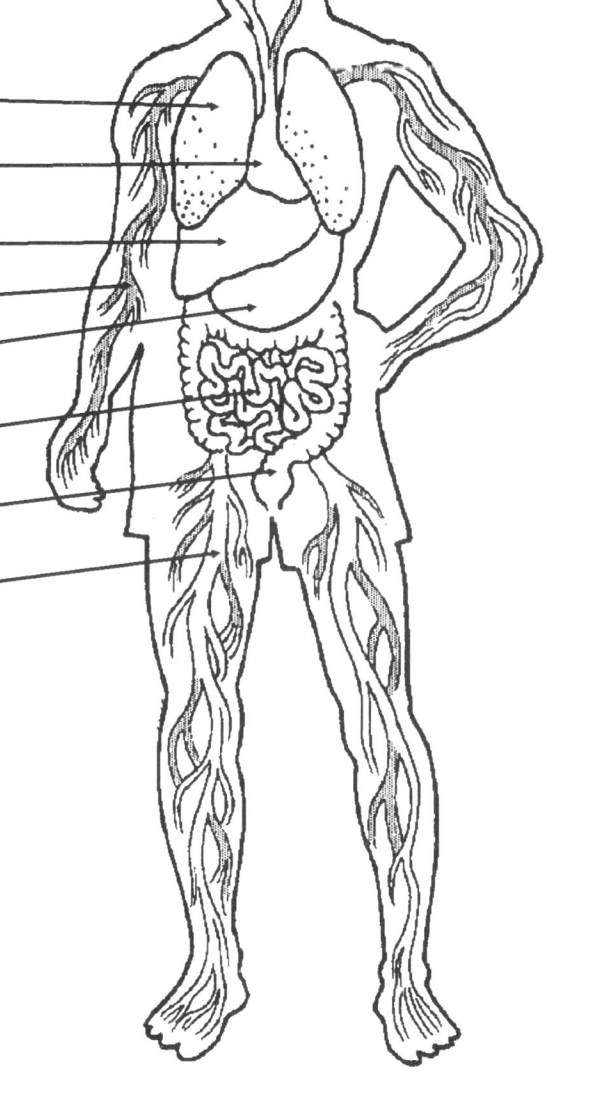

Lesson 2

A Healthy Recipe

Three Bean Salad

1 10-ounce can red kidney beans	1/2 onion
1 10-ounce can corn	1/4 cup light vegetable oil
1 10-ounce can green beans	3 tablespoons vinegar
1 10-ounce can yellow wax beans	1 teaspoon lemon juice
1/2 green pepper	a pinch of salt (to taste)
1 garlic clove	

1. Drain water from the canned beans and corn.

2. Combine corn and beans in a large bowl.

3. Chop onion, green pepper, and garlic into very small pieces.

4. Toss the chopped vegetables with the bean mixture.

5. Mix oil, vinegar, lemon juice, and salt in a small bowl.

6. Pour the dressing over the vegetables and toss. *Makes 6 servings.*

1 2 **3** 4 5 6 7 8

Eat a Variety of Foods

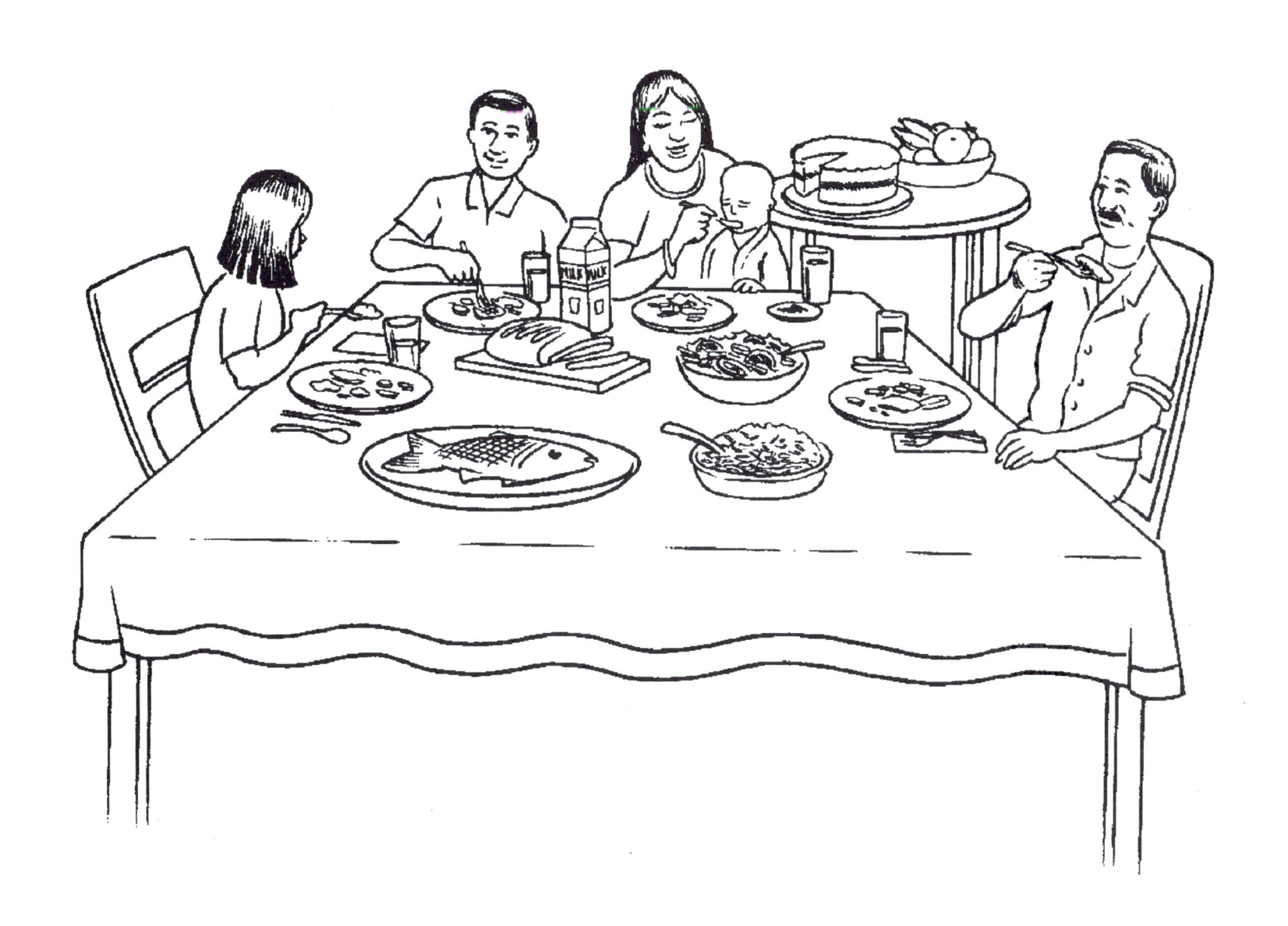

Lesson 3

Your body needs different kinds of foods.

bread, cereal, rice, and pasta

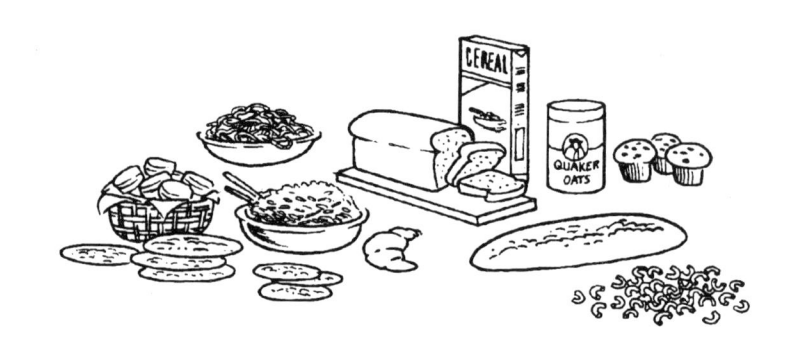

vegetables

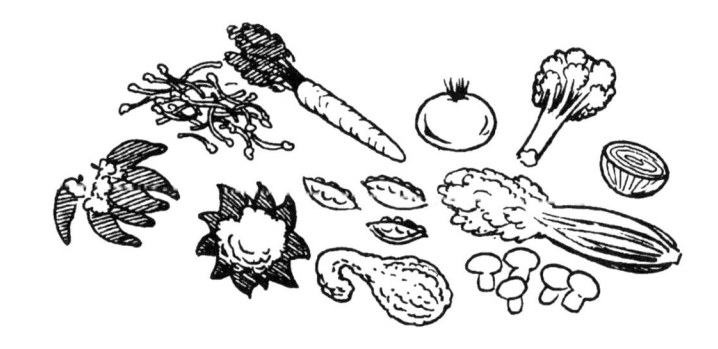

fruit

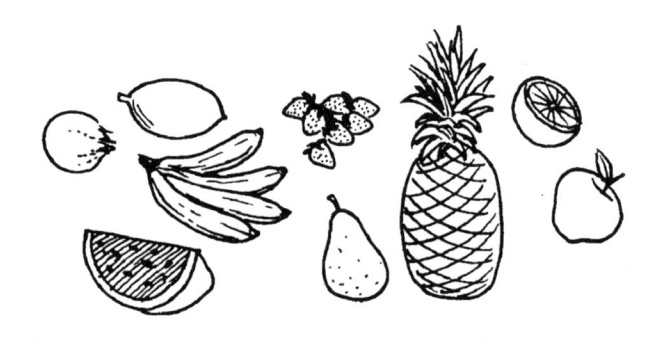

meat, poultry, fish, beans, eggs, and nuts

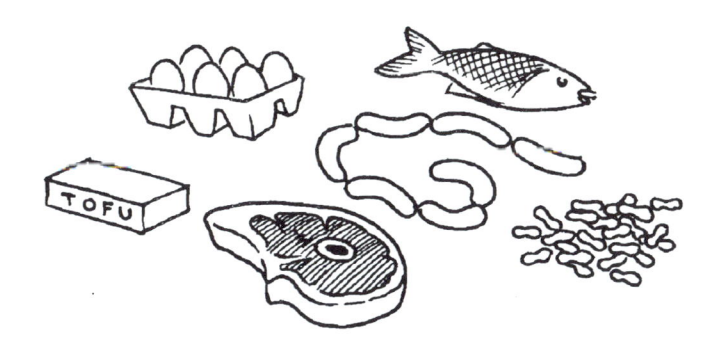

milk, yogurt, and cheese

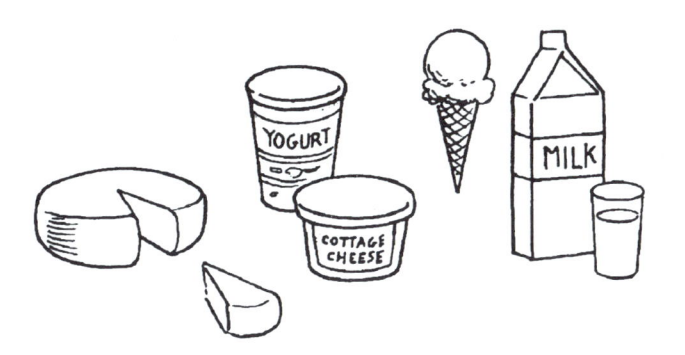

a little fat and oil

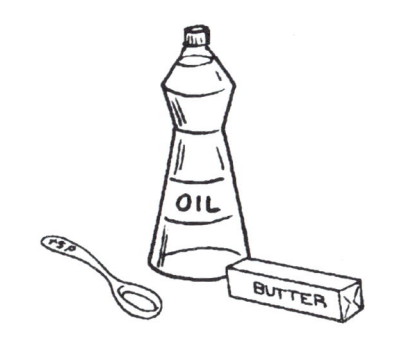

Lesson 3

What do you like to eat?

Hong: What do you like to eat, Maria?

Maria: I like to eat chicken and rice. What do you like to eat, Hong?

Interview your classmates.

Name	grain group	vegetable group	fruit group	milk group	meat group
Maria	rice	carrots	banana	milk	chicken

Your body needs

proteins from the meat group

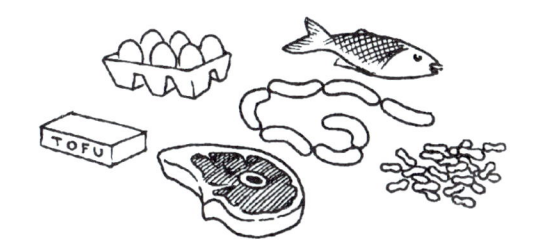

carbohydrates from the grain group

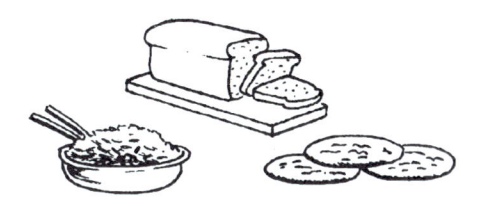

vitamins and minerals from
the vegetable and fruit groups

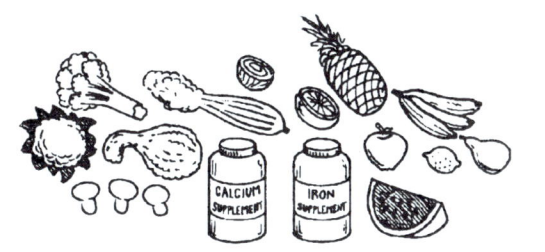

calcium from the milk group

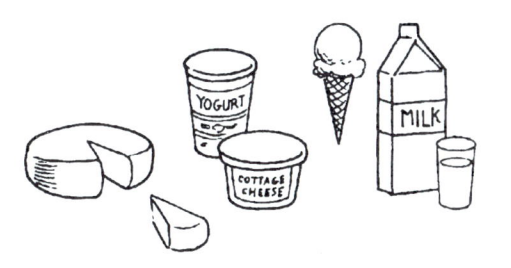

a small amount of fat

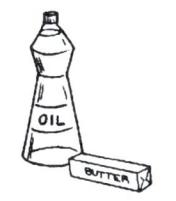

Lesson 3

Circle these words in the label below.

Nutrition Facts

Serving Size 1 cup (228 g)
Servings Per Container 2

Amount Per Serving

Calories 260   Calories from Fat 120

% **Daily Value**

Total Fat 13 g	**20%**
Saturated Fat 5g	**25%**
Cholesterol 30 mg	**10%**
Sodium 660mg	**28%**
Total Carbohydrate 31g	**10%**
Dietary Fiber 0g	**0%**
Sugars 5g	
Protein 5g	

Vitamin A 4%   Vitamin C 2%
Calcium 15%   Iron 4%

carbohydrate

fat

protein

vitamin

calcium

Name foods that have

1. carbohydrates _____

   _____

2. fats _____

   _____

3. protein _____

   _____

4. vitamins and minerals _____

   _____

5. calcium _____

   _____

Lesson 3

Servings

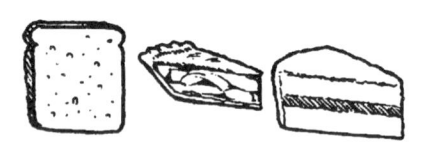

a slice = a piece

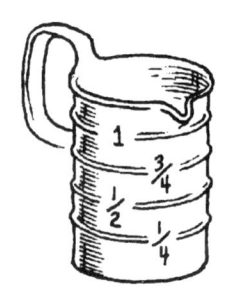

cup = c.

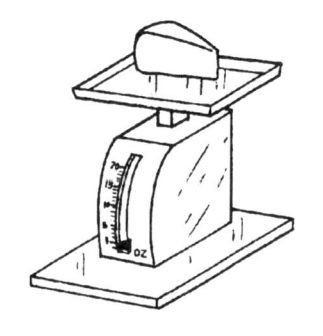

ounce = oz.

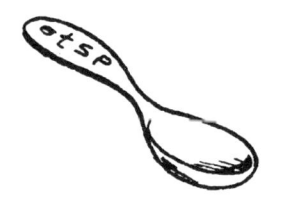

teaspoon = tsp.

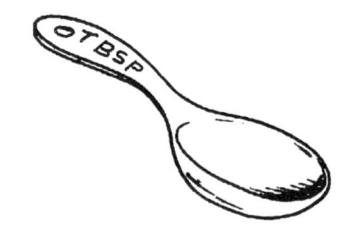

tablespoon = Tbsp.

Fill in the servings.

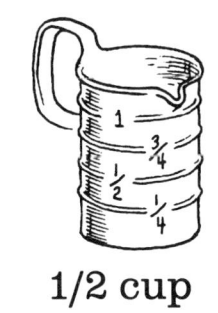

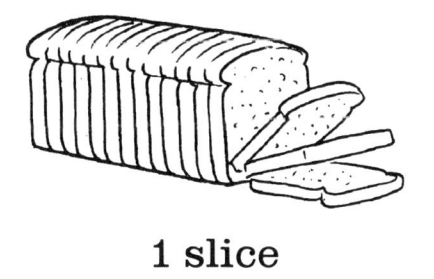

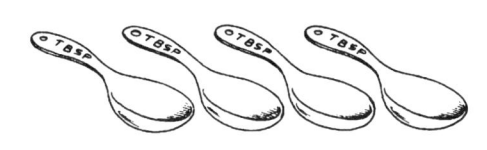

1/2 cup

1 slice

3 Tbsps.

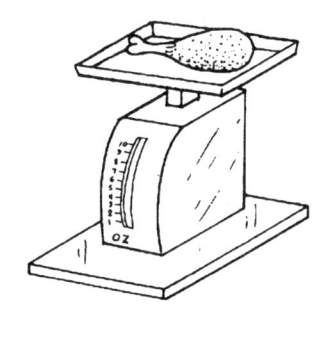

3 oz.

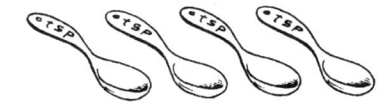

2 tsps.

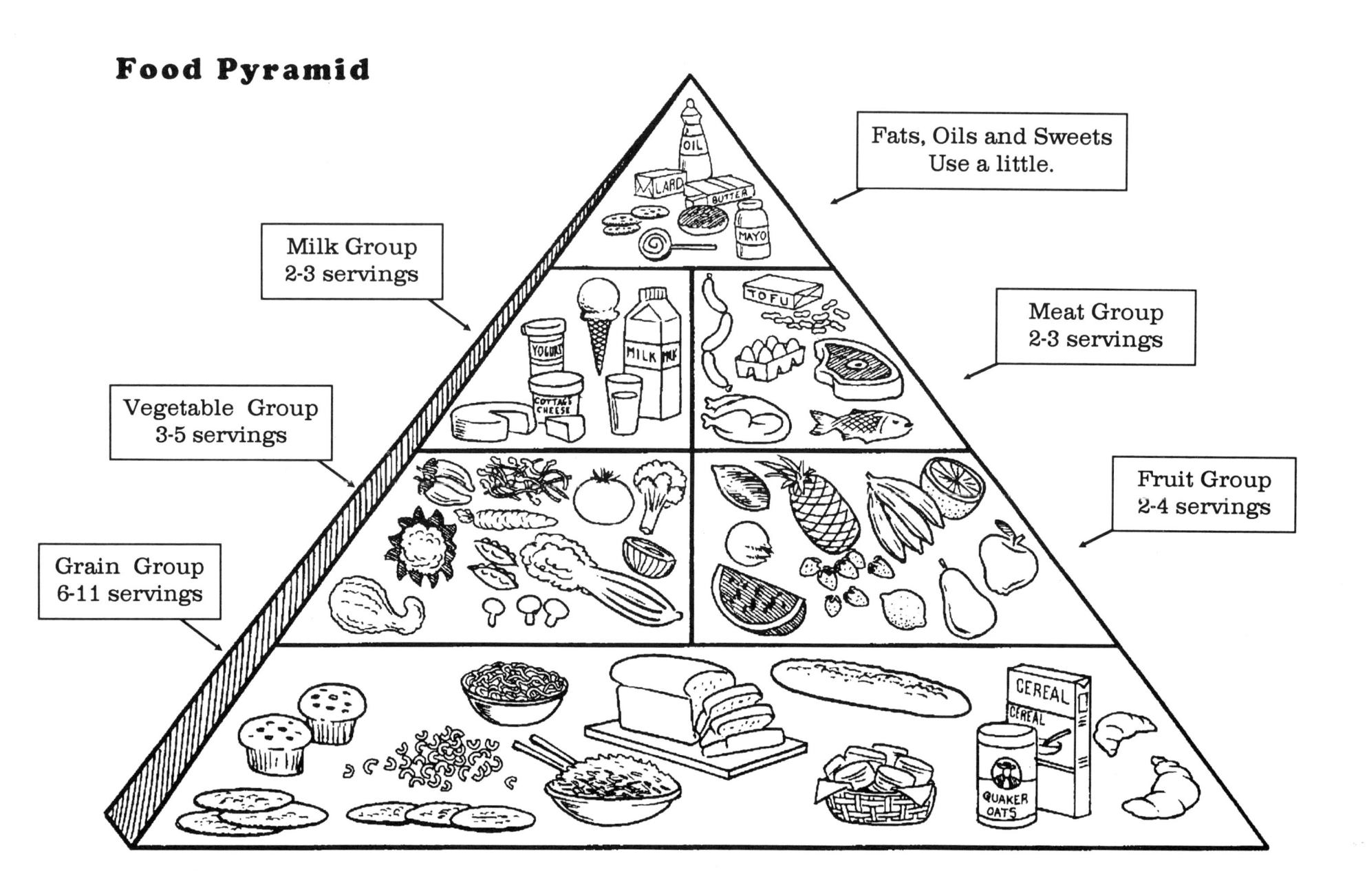

Lesson 3

Food Pyramid

Fats, Oils and Sweets
Use a little.

Milk Group
2-3 servings

Meat Group
2-3 servings

Vegetable Group
3-5 servings

Fruit Group
2-4 servings

Grain Group
6-11 servings

40

What is a serving?

Grain Group	Vegetable Group	Fruit Group	Milk Group	Meat Group
1 slice of bread or 1 tortilla	1 cup of raw vegetables	1 medium apple, banana, orange	1 cup of milk or yogurt	3 ounces of cooked meat, poultry, or fish
1 ounce of cereal	1/2 cup of other vegetables, cooked or chopped raw	1/2 cup of chopped, cooked, or canned fruit	1 1/2 ounces of cheese	1/2 cup of cooked beans, 1 egg, or 2 tablespoons of peanut butter count as 1 ounce of meat
1/2 cup of cooked cereal, rice, or pasta	3/4 cup of vegetable juice	3/4 cup of fruit juice		

Lesson 3

What did you eat yesterday?

Breakfast: _____

_____

Lunch: _____

_____

Dinner: _____

_____

Snacks: _____

_____

Lesson 3

How many servings did you eat yesterday?

(Check one box for each serving.)

Fats, Oils, and Sweets ☐ ☐ ☐ ☐ ☐ ☐ ☐ ☐

Milk Group ■ ■ ■ ☐ ☐ ☐ ☐ ☐

Meat Group ■ ■ ■ ☐ ☐ ☐ ☐ ☐

Fruit Group ■ ■ ■ ■ ☐ ☐ ☐ ☐

Vegetable Group ■ ■ ■ ■ ■ ☐ ☐ ☐

Grain Group ■ ■ ■ ■ ■ ■ ■ ■ ■

I feel awful.

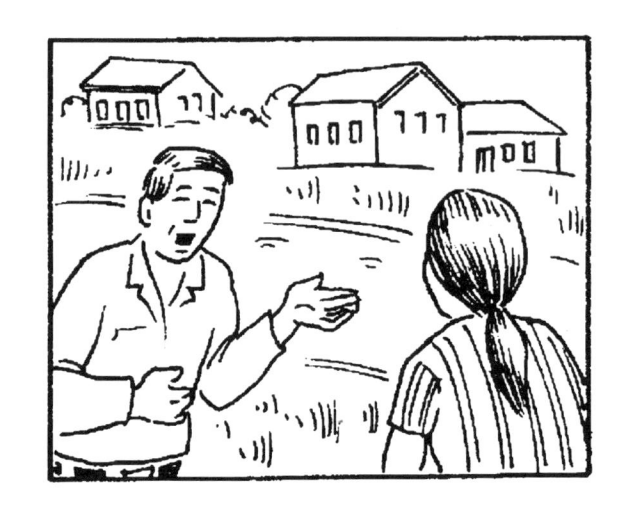

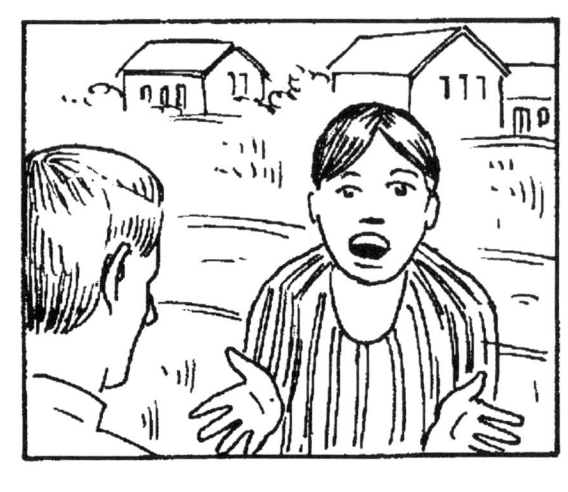

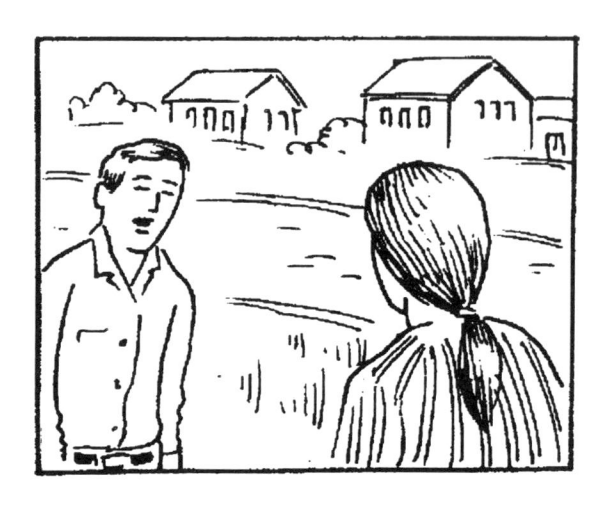

Mary: Hi, Bob. How are you?

Bob: I feel awful. I worked 12 hours today with no lunch break.

Mary: Did you eat anything today?

Bob: Sure. I had a donut for breakfast and french fries and a Coke for dinner.

Answer the questions.

1. How many hours did Bob work today? _____
   _____

2. What did Bob eat? _____
   _____

3. Why does Bob feel awful? _____
   _____

4. What did you eat today? _____
   _____

5. How do you feel? _____
   _____

Lesson 3

A Healthy Recipe

No-Bake Chocolate Oatmeal Cookies

2-4 tablespoons cocoa
2 tablespoons oil
1 teaspoon vanilla
1 cup sugar

1/2 teaspoon salt
1/4 cup milk
1 1/2 cups oatmeal

1. Mix cocoa, sugar, milk, oil, and salt in a saucepan.
2. Boil for 3 minutes. Stir the mixture while it boils.
3. Remove from heat. Stir the oatmeal and vanilla into the mixture.
4. Place spoonfuls onto a cookie sheet or large plate.
5. The cookies are ready to eat when they are cool and hard. *Makes 2 dozen cookies.*

1 2 3 **4** 5 6 7 8

Make Healthy Meals

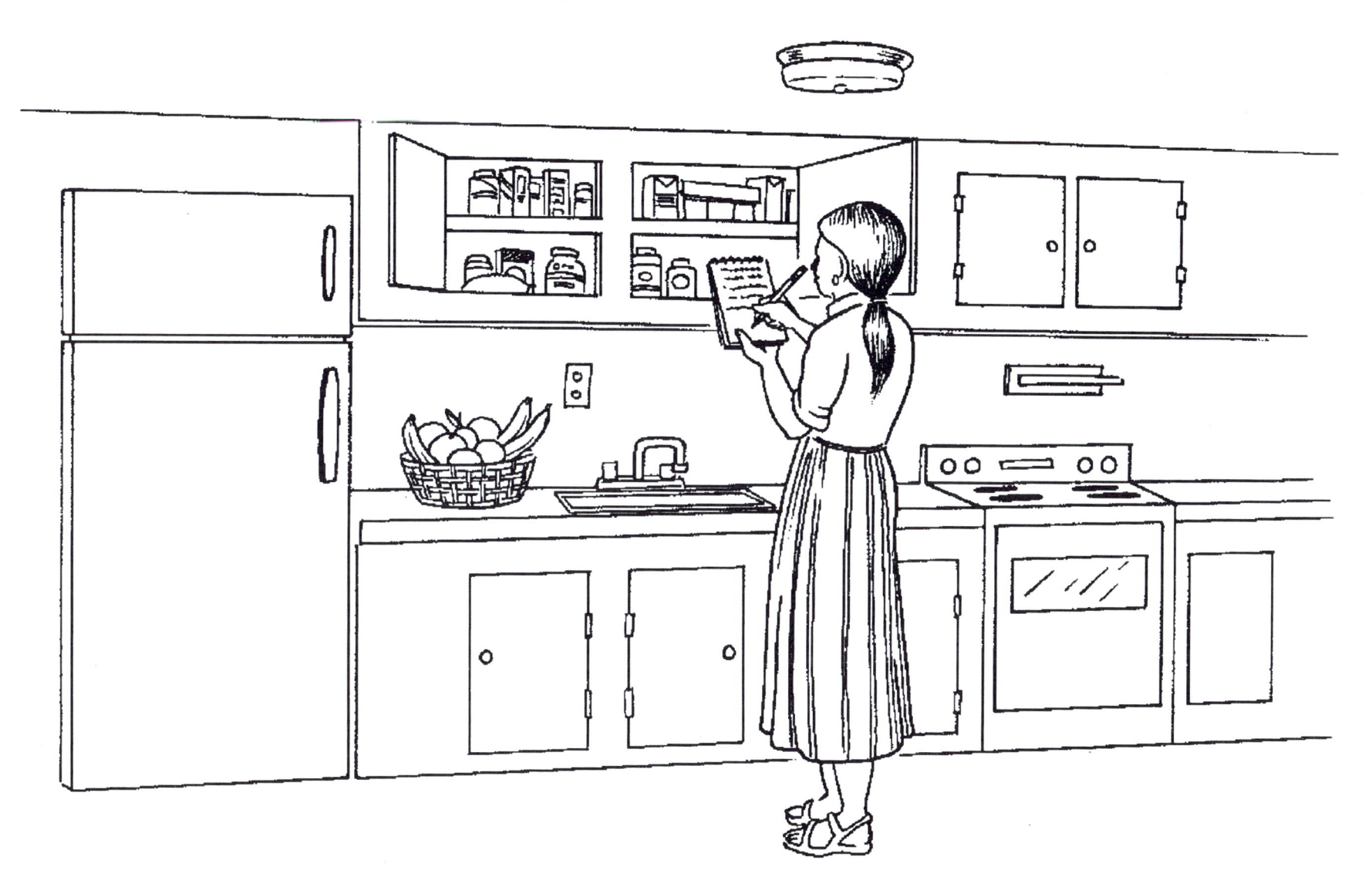

Lesson 4

Name the food groups.

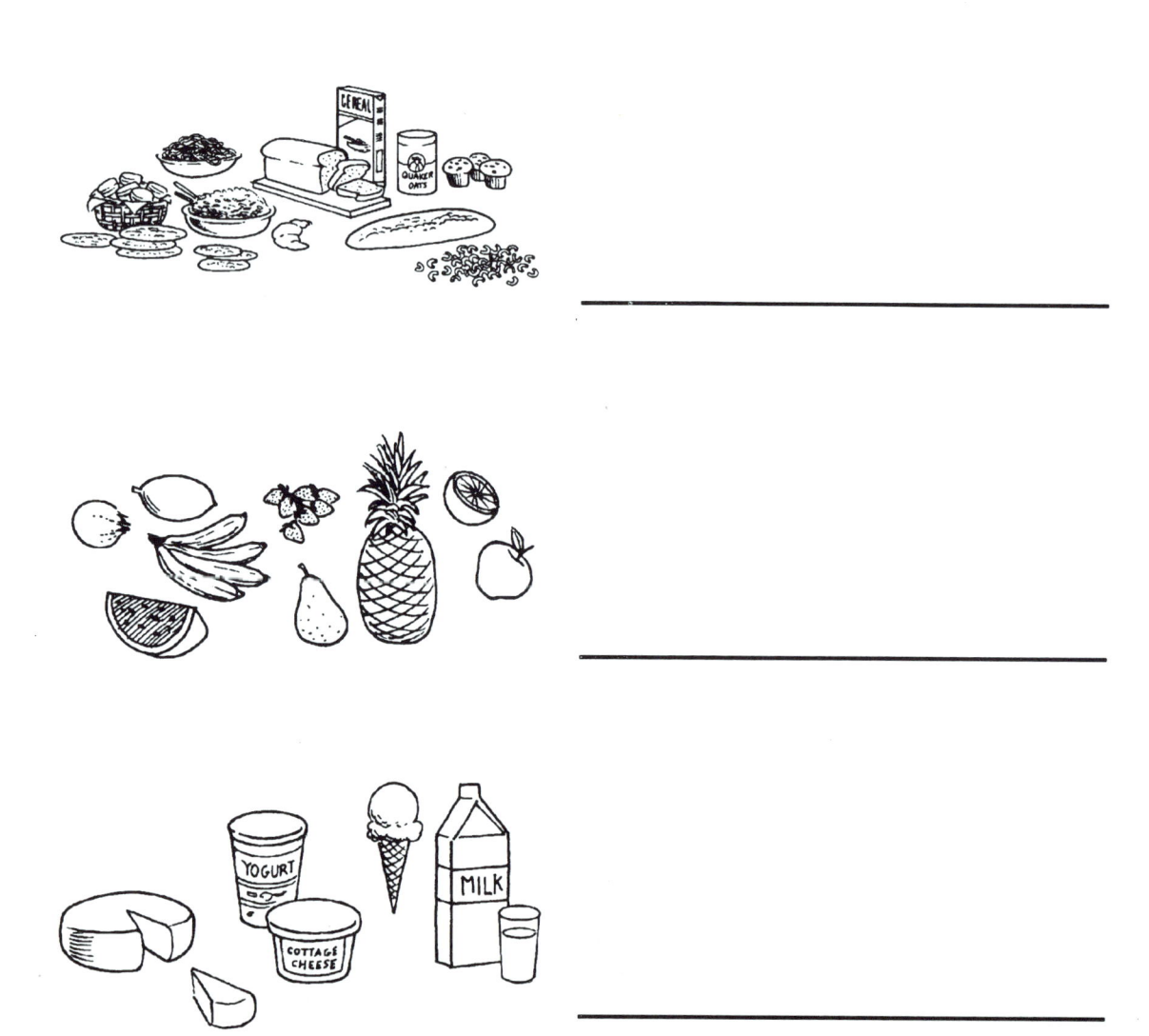

_____

_____

_____

Lesson 4

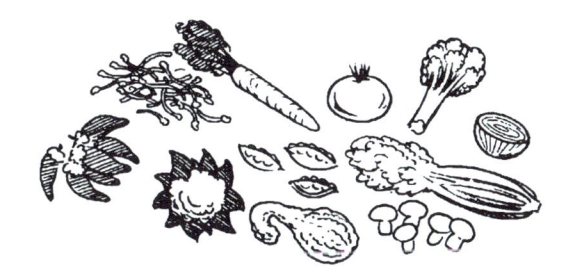

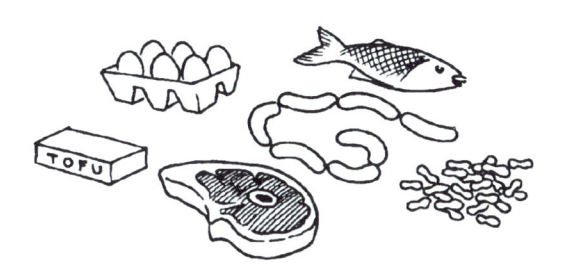

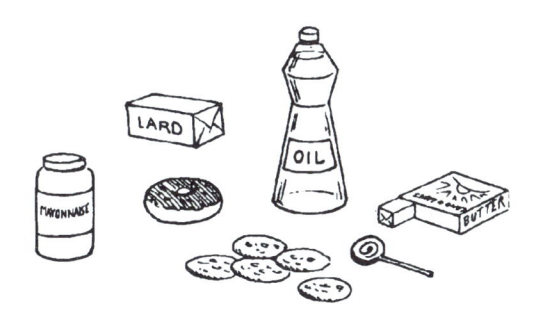

_____

_____

_____

Meat Group

Fruit Group

Grain Group

Fats, Oils and Sweets

Vegetable Group

Milk Group

Lesson 4

Plan a healthy meal.

Plan a meal using all of the food groups.

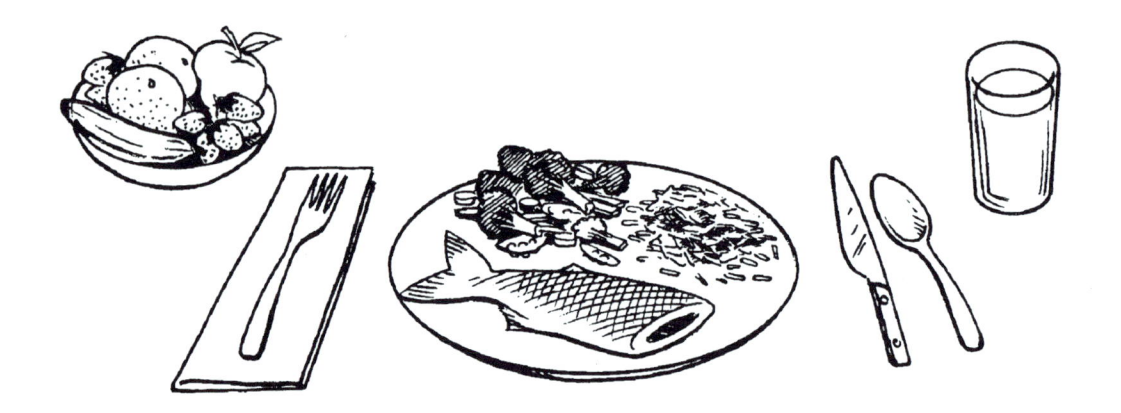

Plan your meal.

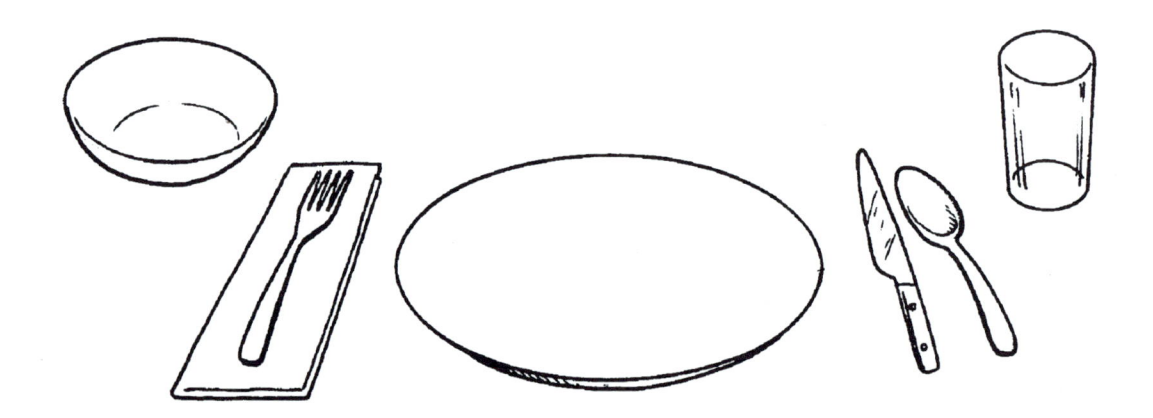

Better Than Meat

A grain with a legume gives your body the same energy as the meat group.

Grains + Legumes = Meat Group

Rice + Beans = Meat Group

🍚 + 🫘 = Meat Group

Rice + Tofu = Meat Group

🍚 + TOFU = Meat Group

Bread + Peanut Butter = Meat Group

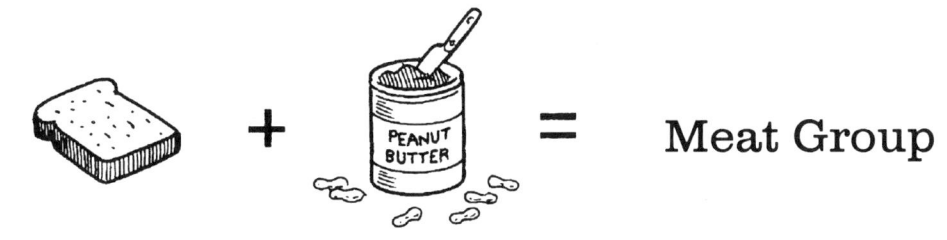

🍞 + PEANUT BUTTER = Meat Group

Lesson 4

Which is healthier for you?

1.

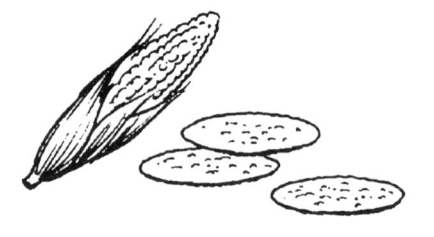

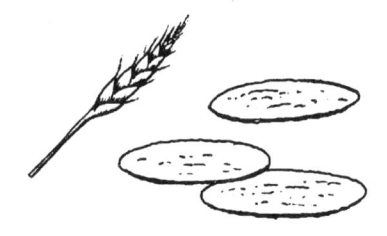

corn tortilla   flour tortilla

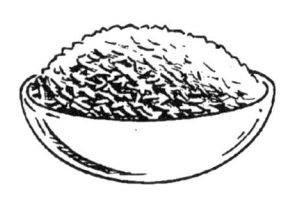

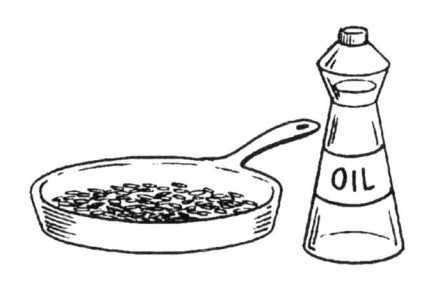

2.

rice   rice and oil

Lesson 4

3.

fruit juice   cola

4.

donuts   bread

5.

dried fish   fresh fish

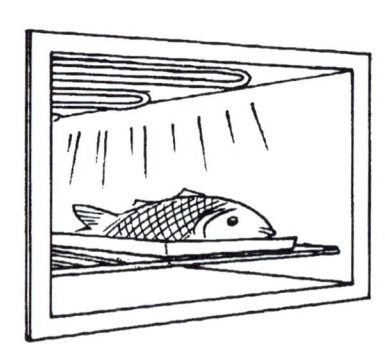

Lesson 4

Cook foods the healthy way.

bake or roast

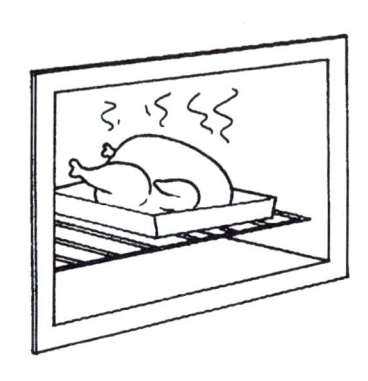

broil

steam

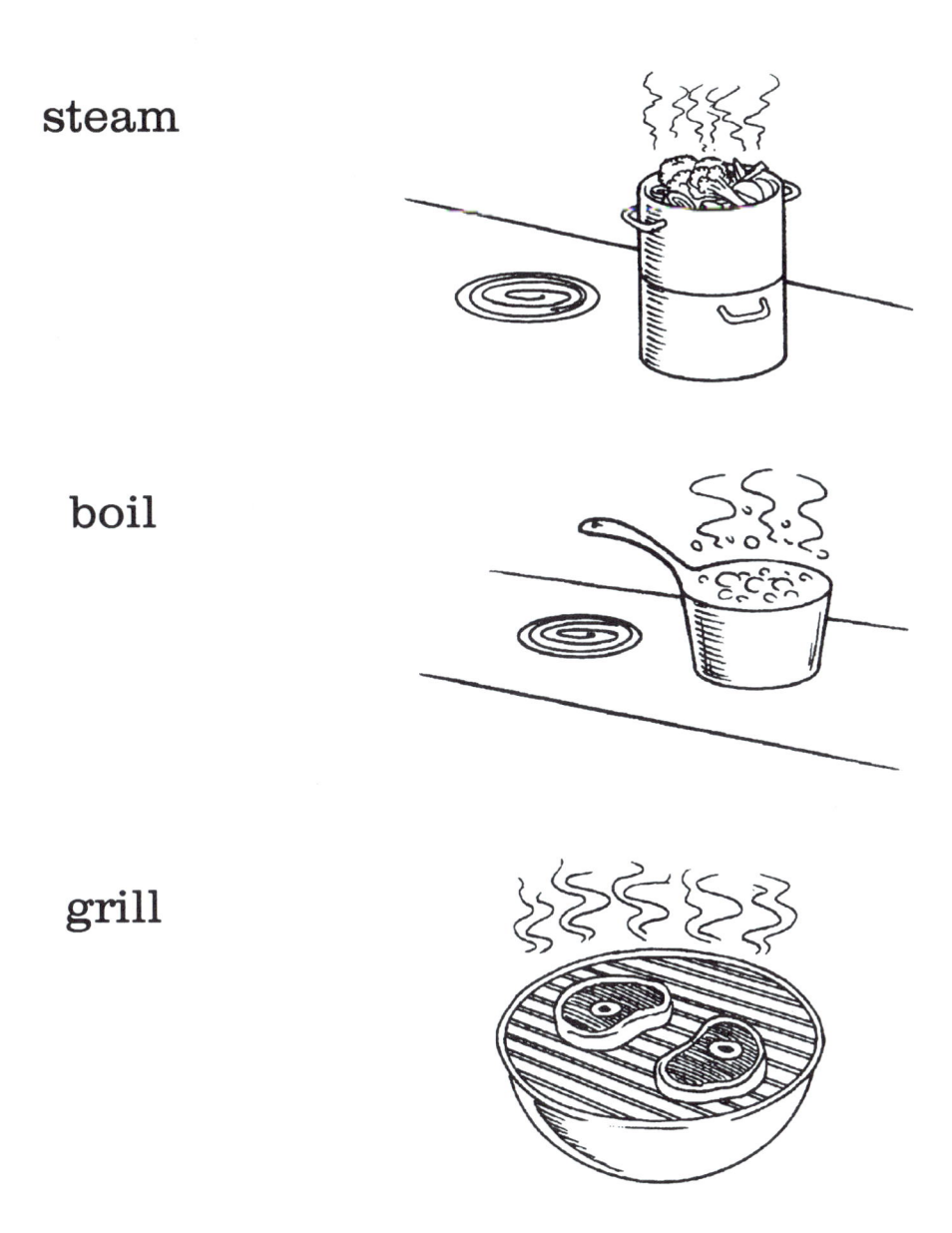

boil

grill

Lesson 4

Cook with less salt.

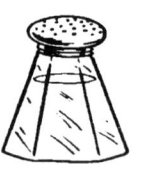

Do not add salt to rice, noodles, or hot cereals.

Canned soup, vegetables, and cheeses have salt in them already.
Do not add more salt.

Soy sauce, onion salt, garlic salt, meat tenderizer and MSG are high in sodium. Use only a little.

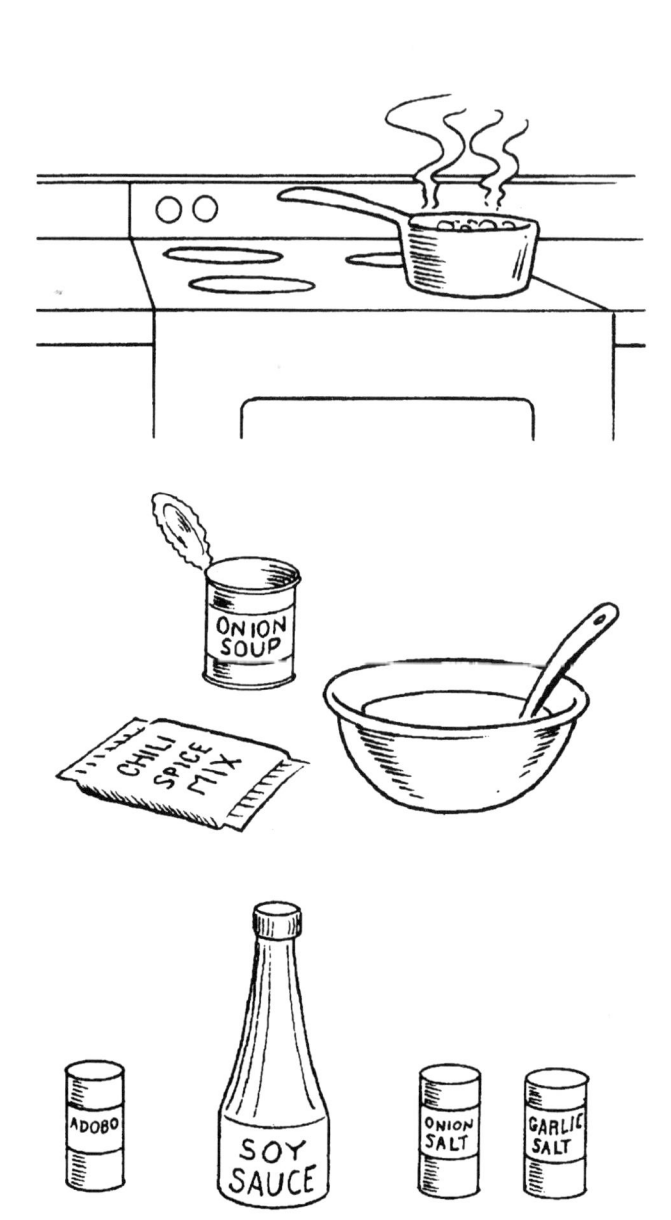

Add spices to make food taste good.

	basil	curry powder	garlic	ginger	oregano	rosemary
chicken			X			X
tomatoes	X				X	
rice	X	X		X		
broccoli		X				
green beans						X
peas						X

Buy foods that are "low sodium," "reduced sodium," or "no salt added."

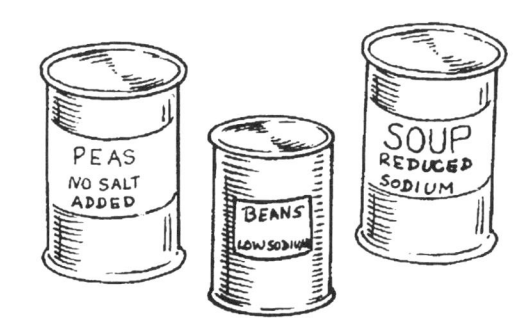

Lesson 4

Cook with less fat.

Cut fat off meat.

Bake, broil, and steam foods.

Use small amounts of oil or margarine in cooking.
Use vegetable spray to fry.

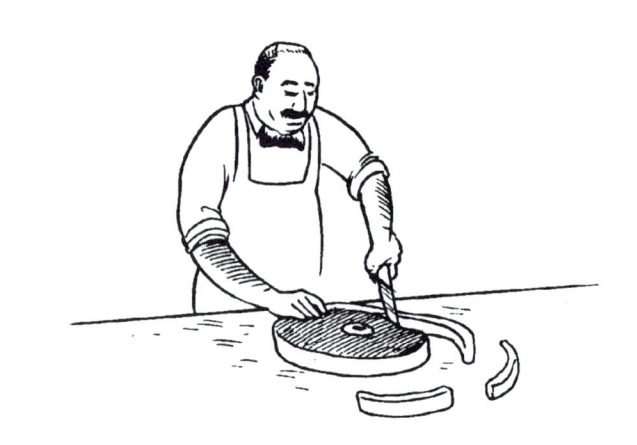

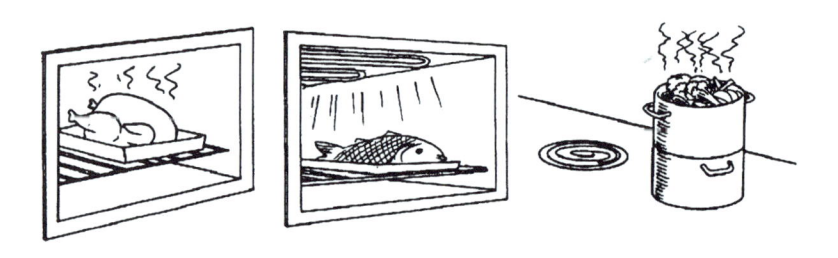

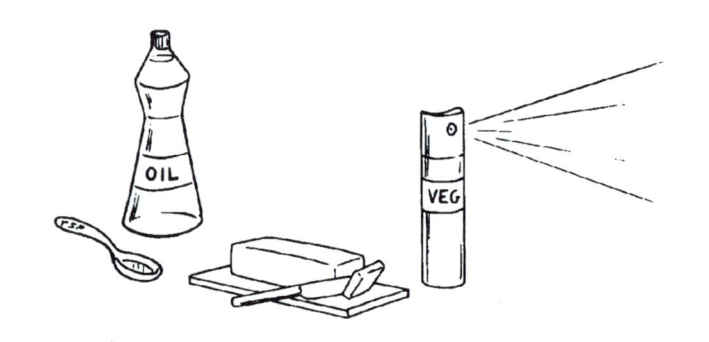

Use lowfat milk or skim milk in recipes.

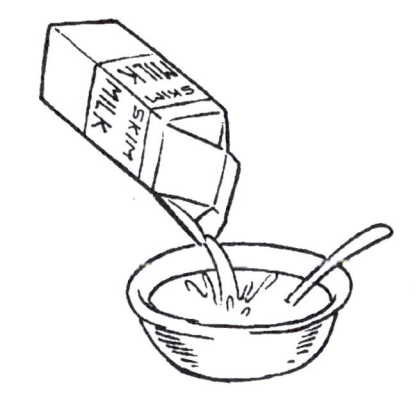

Use lowfat yogurt or lowfat cottage cheese for sour cream or mayonnaise.

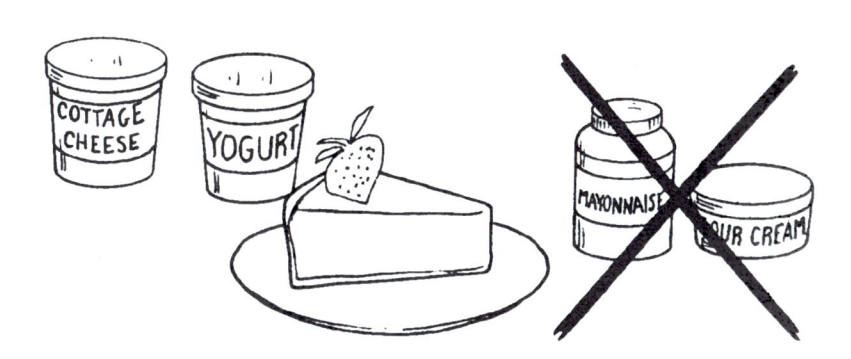

Cool meat broth. Spoon off fat.
Use broth in recipe.

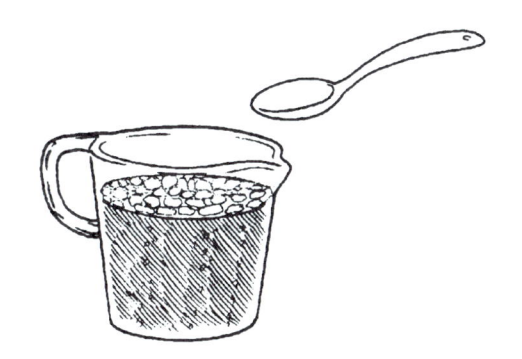

Lesson 4

The Price of a Healthy Meal

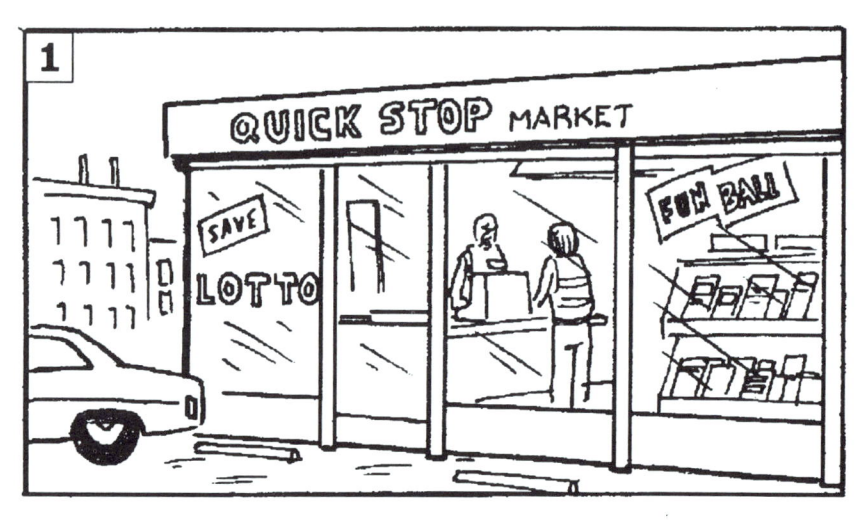

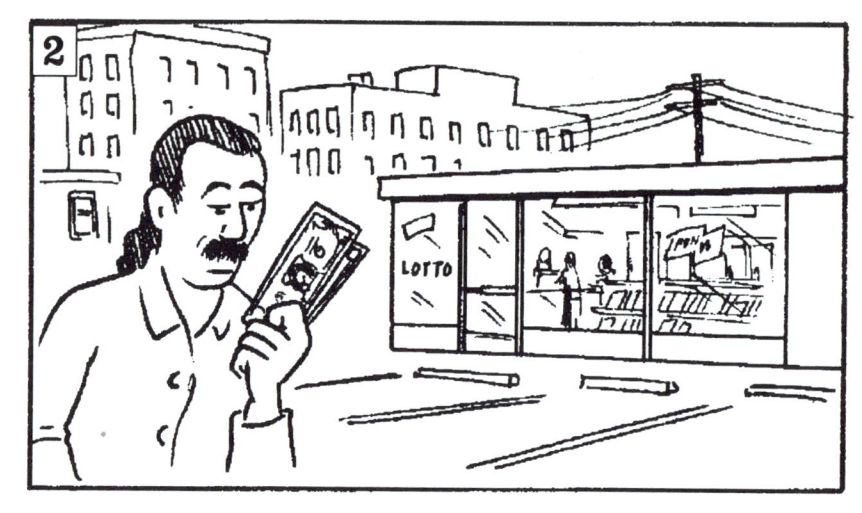

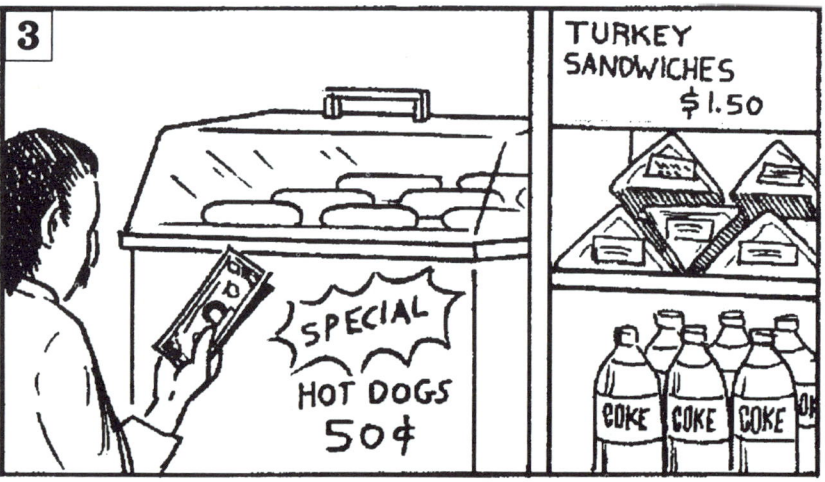

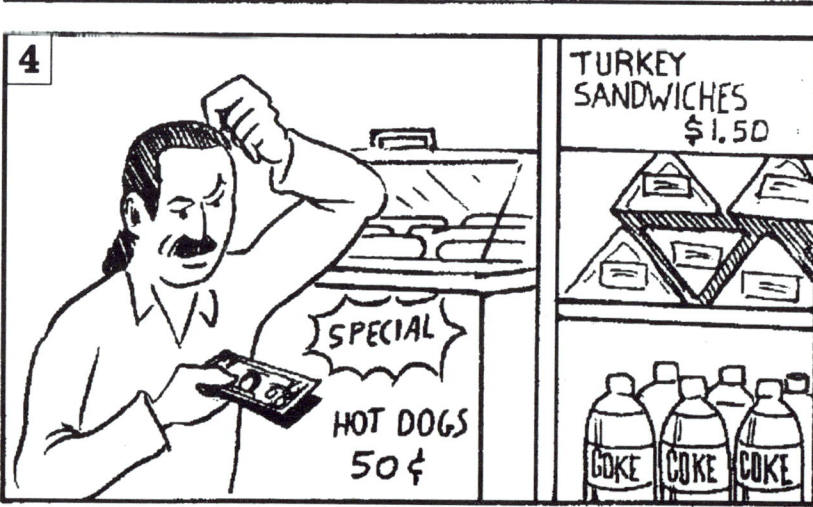

Answer the questions.

1. Where is the man?_____

2. What does the man want?_____

3. What is the problem?_____

4. What will the man do?_____

5. What would you do? _____

Lesson 4

A Healthy Recipe

Banana Milkshake

1/3 cup non-fat dry milk

1 cup water

1 banana

1/2 teaspoon vanilla

1. Mash the banana well.

2. Add milk, water, and vanilla and blend with a beater or shake in a jar.

3. Serve immediately or refrigerate and serve later. *Makes 1 serving.*

1 2 3 4 **5** 6 7 8

Keep Foods Safe

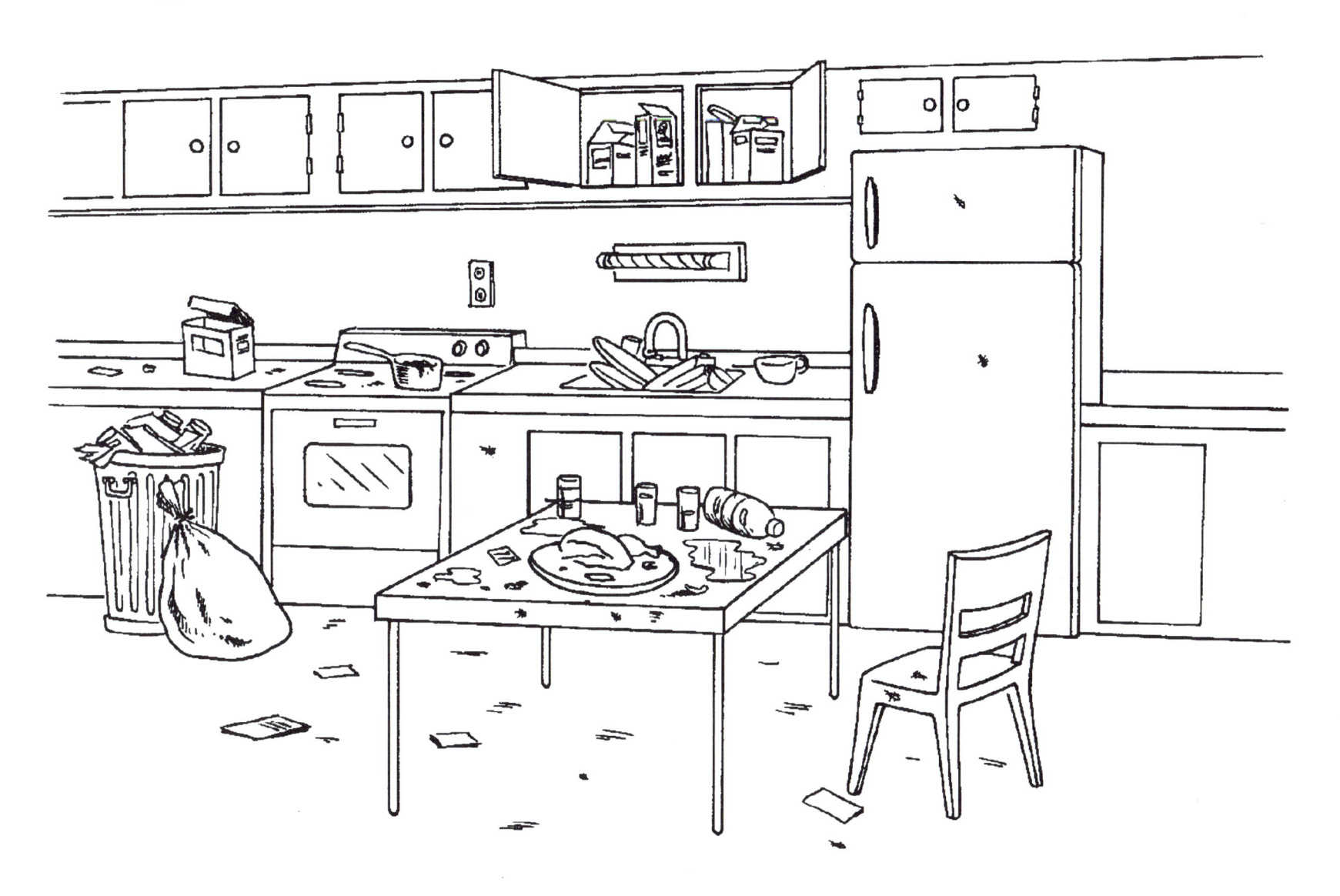

Containers

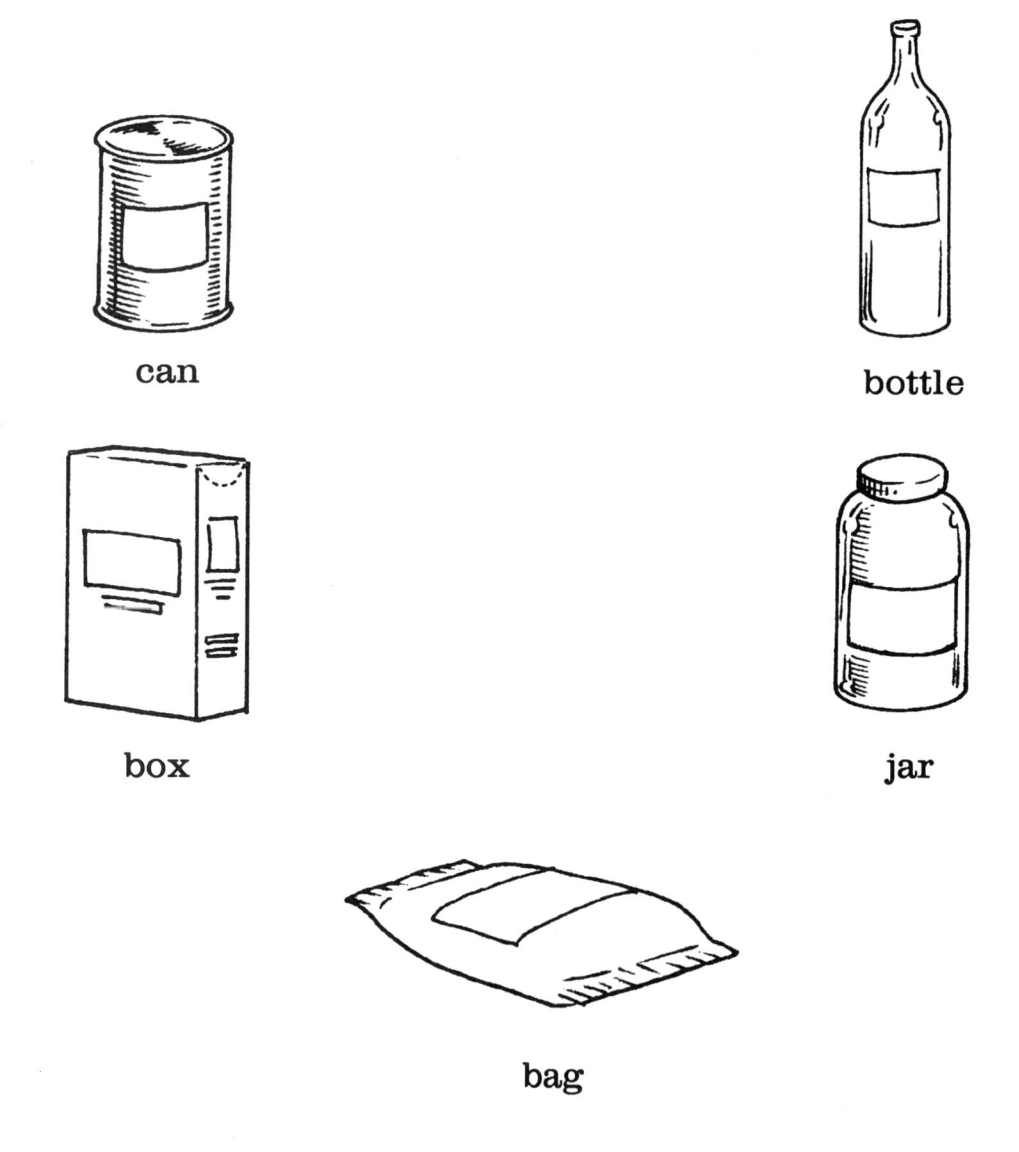

can

bottle

box

jar

bag

Food in the grocery store is ...

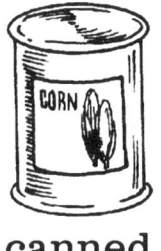

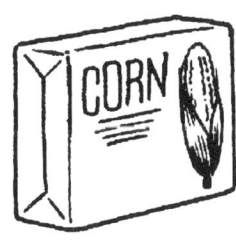

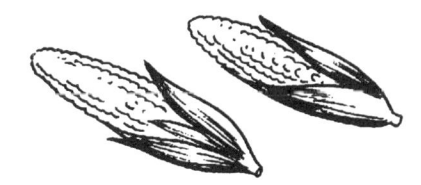

canned   frozen   fresh

Follow the directions.

1. Draw an X through the can.

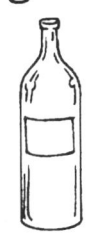

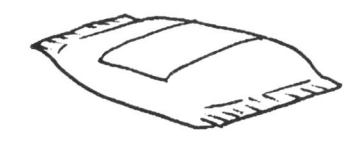

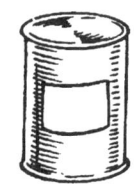

2. Circle the jar.

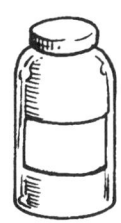

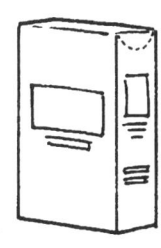

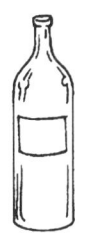

Lesson 5

3. Draw a line under the bag.

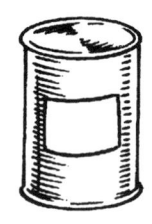

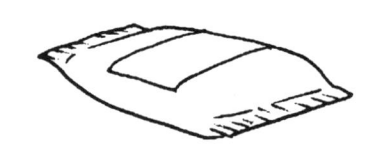

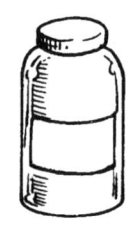

4. Draw an X through the fresh food.

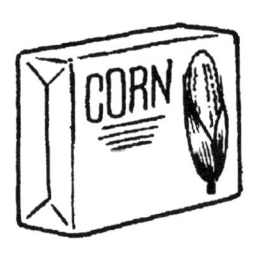

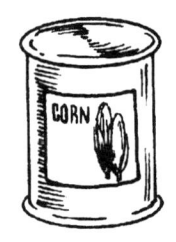

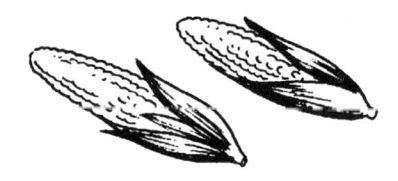

5. Circle the frozen food.

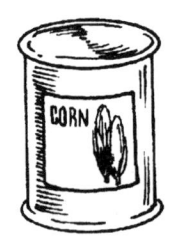

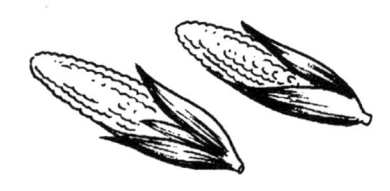

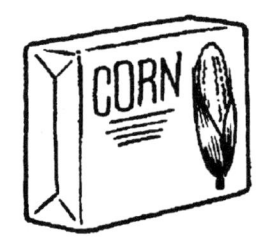

Expiration date

Hamburger		
Total	Per Lb.	Wt.
$2.00	$1.00	2

June 4

Circle the expiration date.

Chicken		
10/15/94		
Total	Per Lb.	Wt.
$2.97	$.99	3

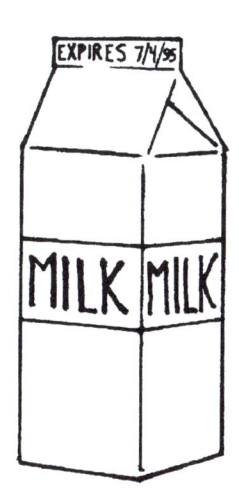

EXPIRES 7/4/95

MILK

Lesson 5

How long can you keep food?

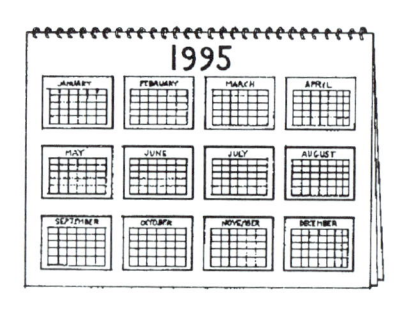

Foods	Shelf	Refrigerator	Freezer
Canned			
soup	1 year		
beans	1 year		
Fresh			
chicken		1-2 days	9-12 months
hamburger		1-2 days	3-4 months
Cooked			
beef		3-4 days	2-3 months
chicken		2-3 days	4-6 months

Circle True (T) or False (F).

1. Fresh hamburger is good for 9-12 months in the refrigerator. T F

2. Cooked chicken is good for 4-6 months in the freezer. T F

3. Canned beans are good for 3 years on the shelf. T F

4. Fresh chicken is good for 3-4 months in the freezer. T F

5. Cooked beef is good for 3-4 days in the refrigerator. T F

Lesson 5

Refrigerator Temperature

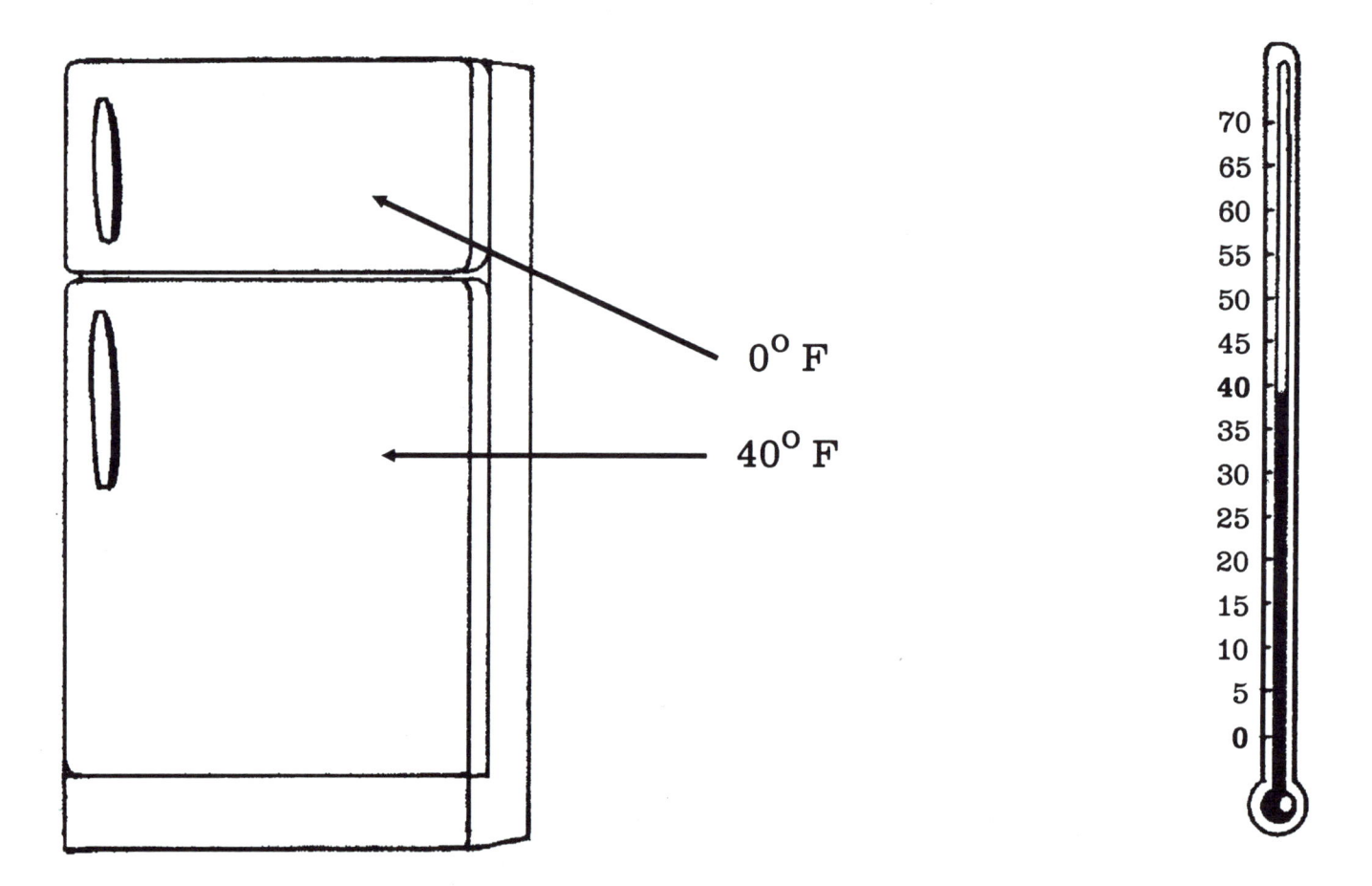

0° F

40° F

Keep your refrigerator at 40° F (4° C). Keep your freezer at 0° F (-18° C).

Don't get sick.

Keep hot foods hot. Keep cold foods cold.

Always cook food completely.

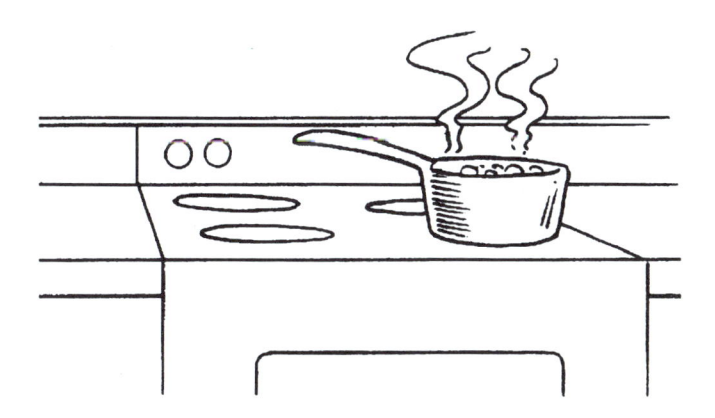

Always thaw frozen food
in the refrigerator.

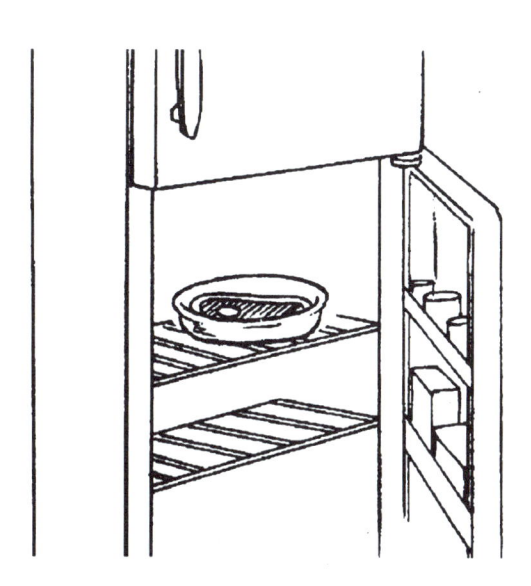

Lesson 5

Always cover and put leftovers in the refrigerator immediately.

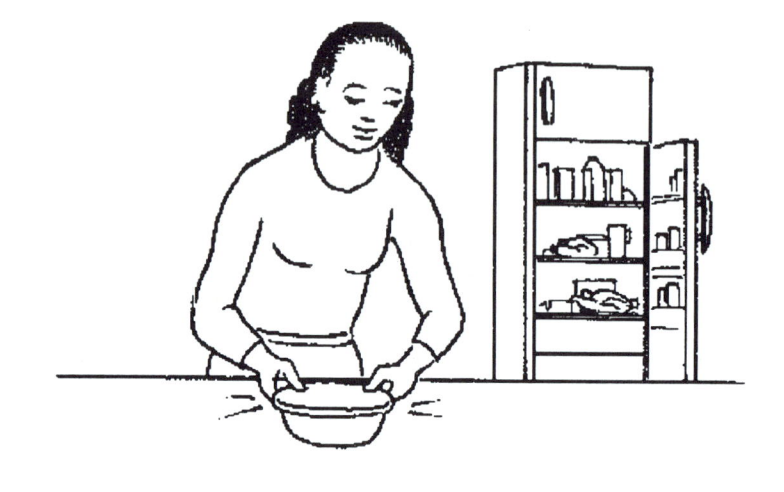

Never buy cracked jars or bulging cans.

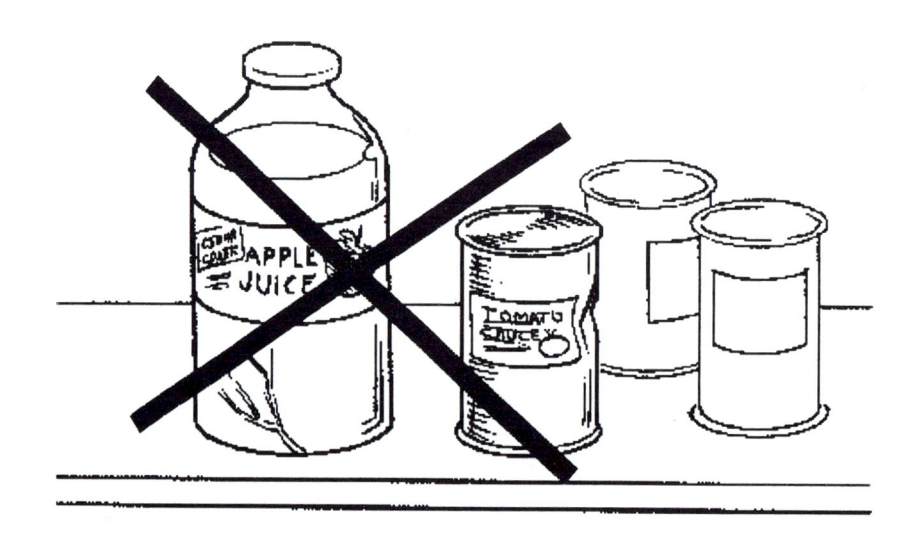

Lesson 5

Never eat raw eggs.

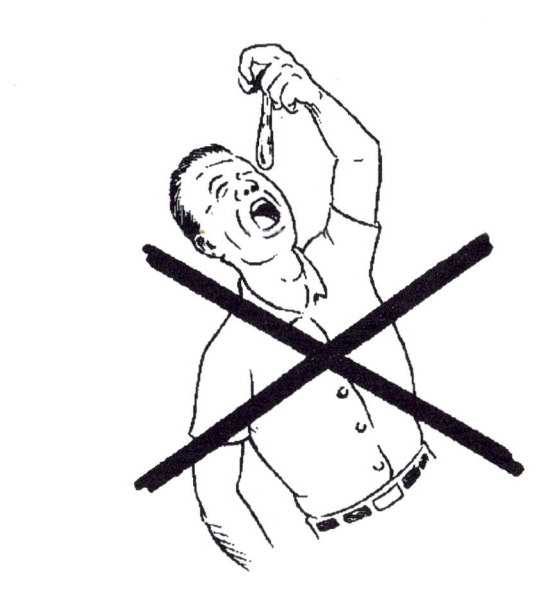

Never keep leftovers on the stove.

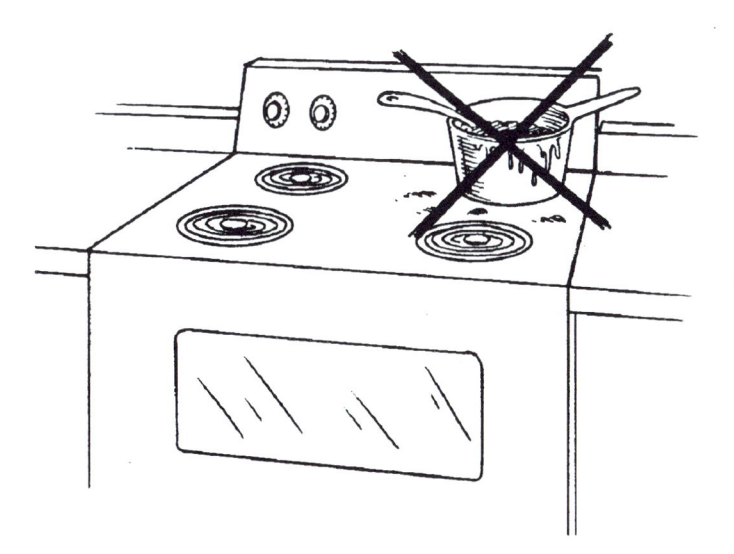

Lesson 5

Keep your hands and utensils clean.

Wash your hands with soap before cooking.

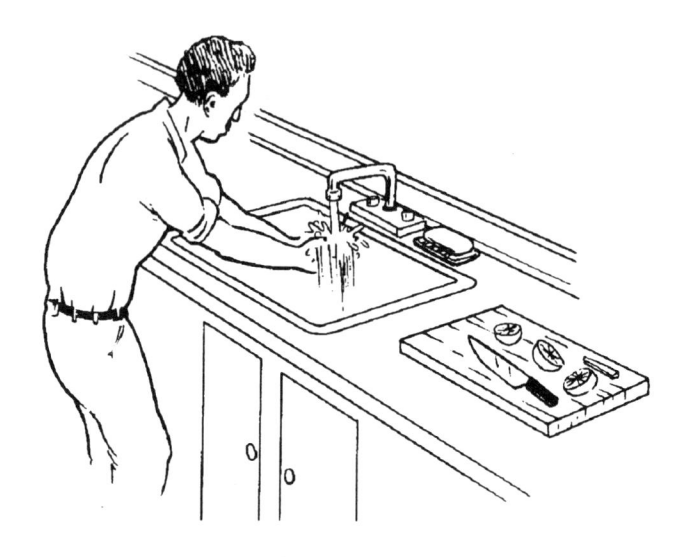

Wash your dishes after eating.

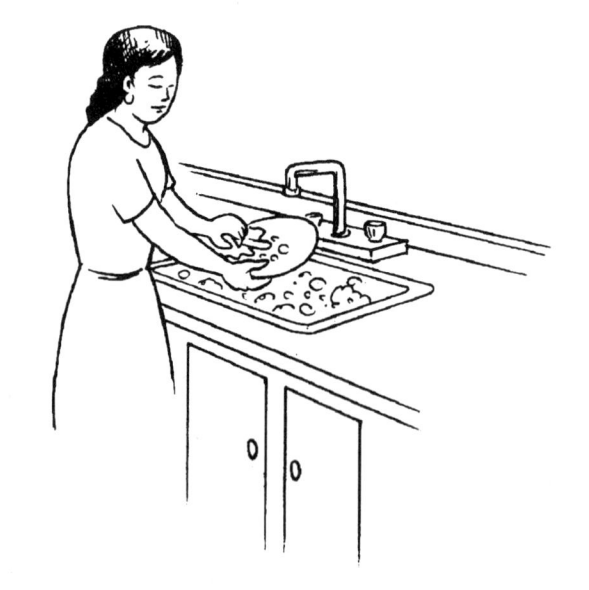

Air dry your dishes after washing.

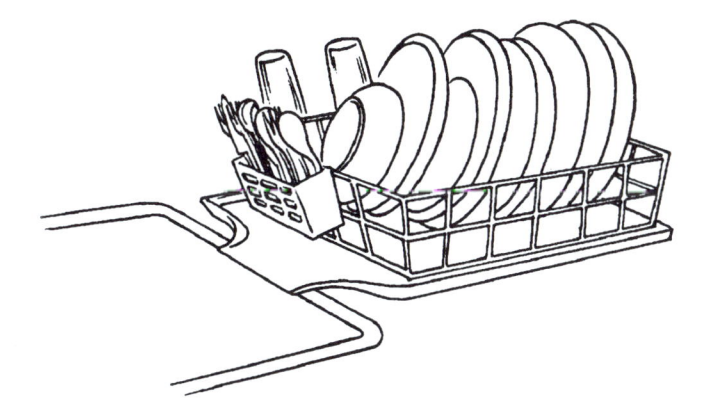

Wash countertops and cutting boards.

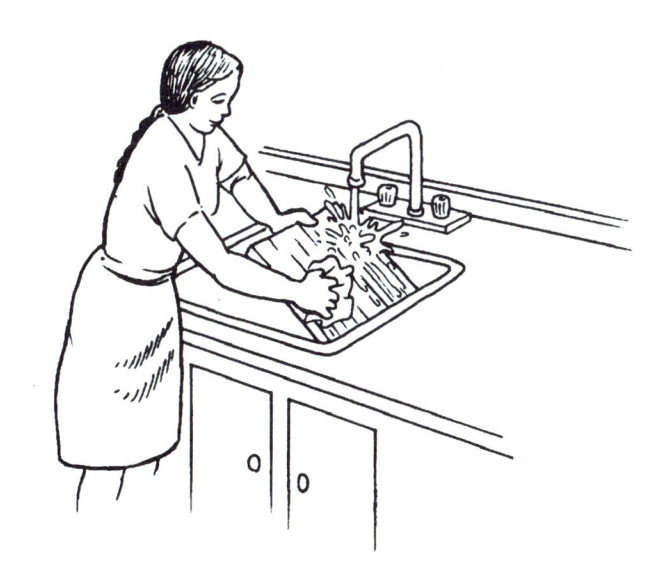

Lesson 5

Keep pests away.

Use fly paper or pest strips
to get rid of flies.

Roaches often live in brown grocery bags.
Keep bags away from the kitchen.

Keep garbage away from the house.
Cover garbage cans.

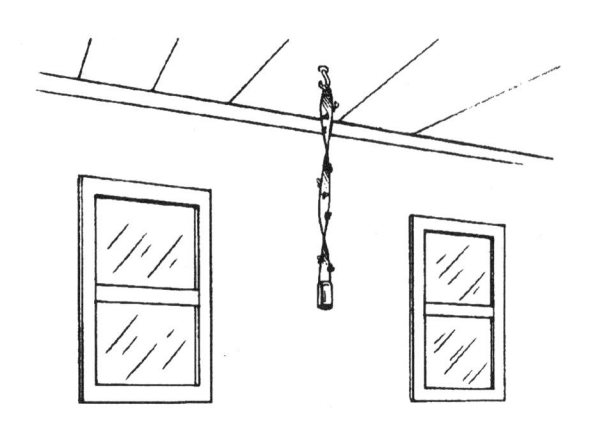

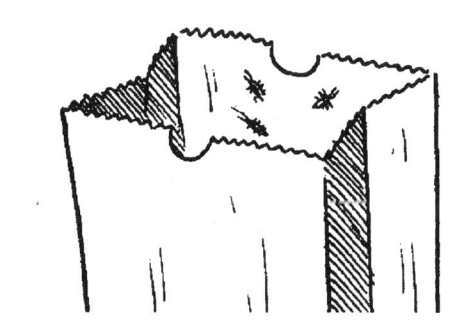

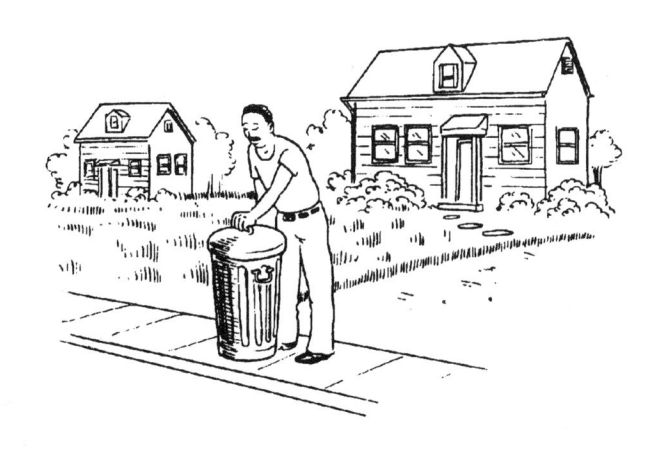

Make a check under your answer.

	always	sometimes	never
1. Do you keep meat, eggs and leftovers in the refrigerator?			
2. Do you thaw your food in the refrigerator?			
3. Do you wash your hands with soap before cooking?			
4. Do you wash your dishes after eating?			
5. Do you air dry your dishes?			
6. Do you wash countertops and cutting boards?			
7. Is your house free of flies and roaches?			

Lesson 5

A Healthy Recipe

Fruit Lover's Popsicles

1 cup nonfat dry milk

5 cups cold water

1 12-ounce can frozen unsweetened orange juice

1. Mix water with milk powder.

2. Add frozen juice.

3. Blend in blender or stir well to blend.

4. Pour into 14 paper cups

5. Cover each paper cup with a square of foil.

6. Use a knife to make a slit in the center of each foil top.

7. Push a wooden popsicle stick through the hole and into the juice mixture.

8. Put the popsicles in the freezer for about 6 hours or until firm. *Makes 14 servings.*

1 2 3 4 5 **6** 7 8

Be a Smart Shopper

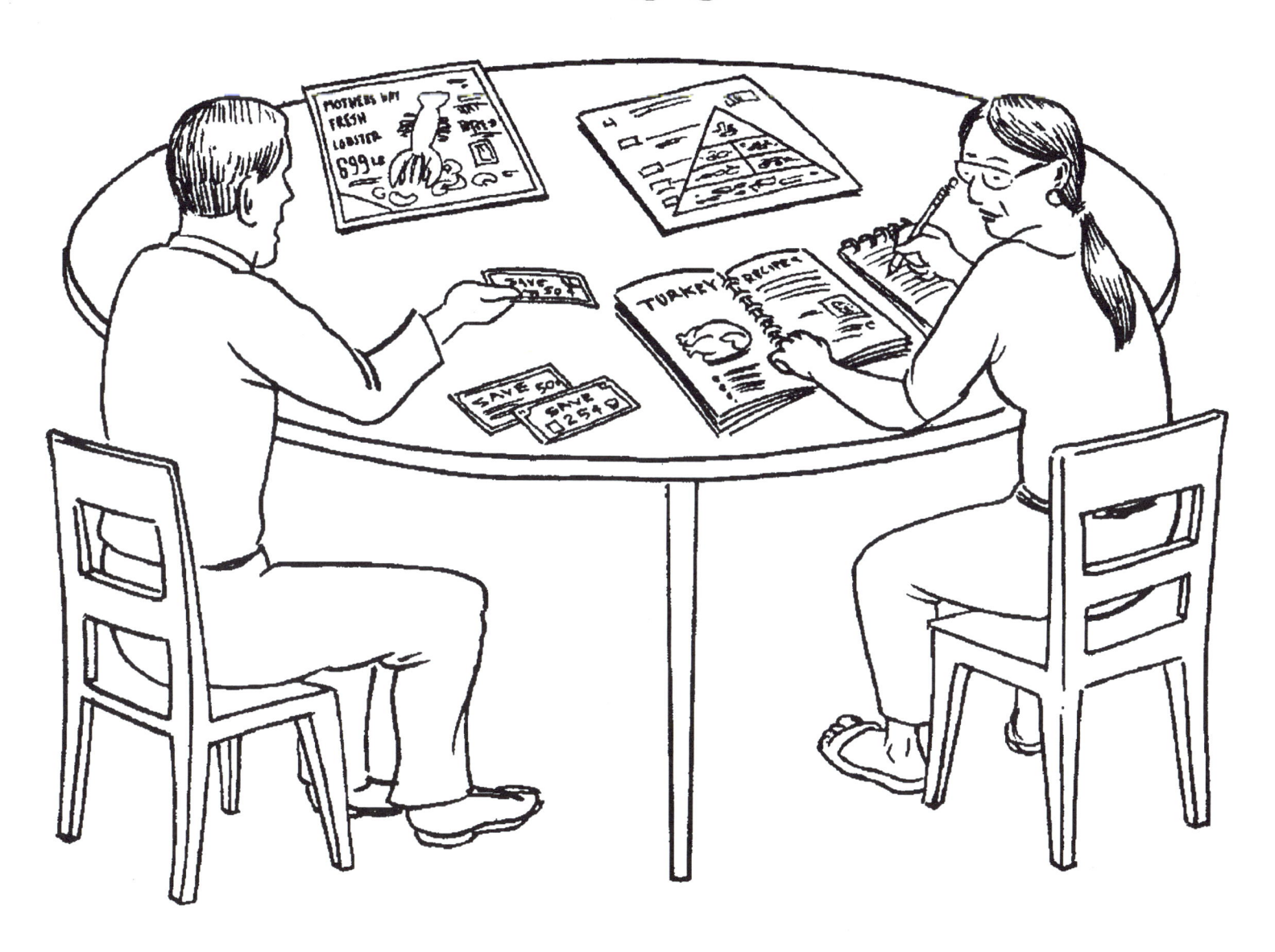

Lesson 6

Look for specials.

Meat and Poultry

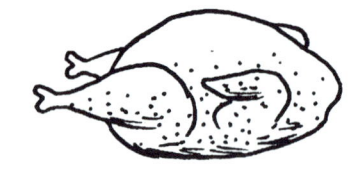

fresh roaster .69¢ lb.

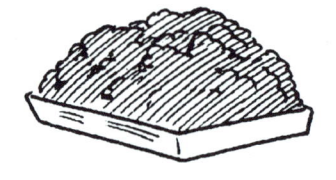

fresh ground beef $1.69 lb.

Fresh Produce

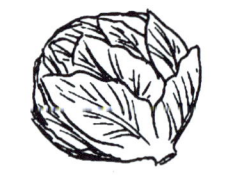

lettuce .79¢ each

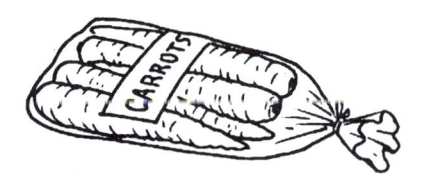

carrots 2 lb. bag .79¢

Bakery

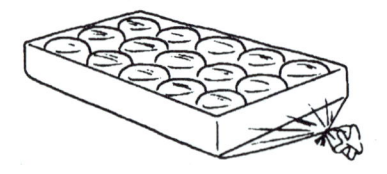

dinner rolls .99¢
package of 12

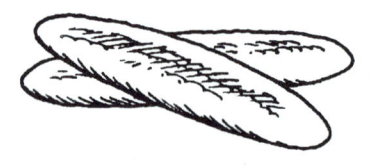

bread .79¢ loaf

Frozen Foods

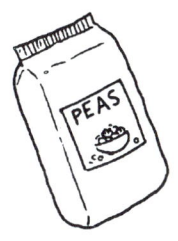

frozen green peas .99¢
16 oz. package

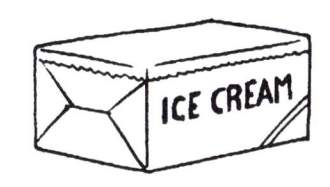

ice cream $1.99
1/2 gallon

1. How much is lettuce? _____

2. How much is a carton of ice cream? _____

3. How much is a pound of ground beef? _____

4. Are these prices expensive? _____

5. Where do you shop? Why?_____

Lesson 6

Find the unit price.

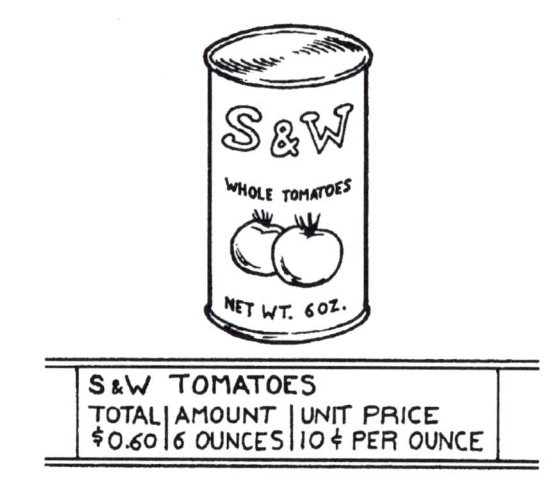

S&W TOMATOES		
TOTAL	AMOUNT	UNIT PRICE
$0.60	6 OUNCES	10¢ PER OUNCE

1. How much is one ounce of tomatoes? _____

2. What's the total price? _____

3. What's the total weight? _____

4. What's the brand name of the food? _____

Lesson 6

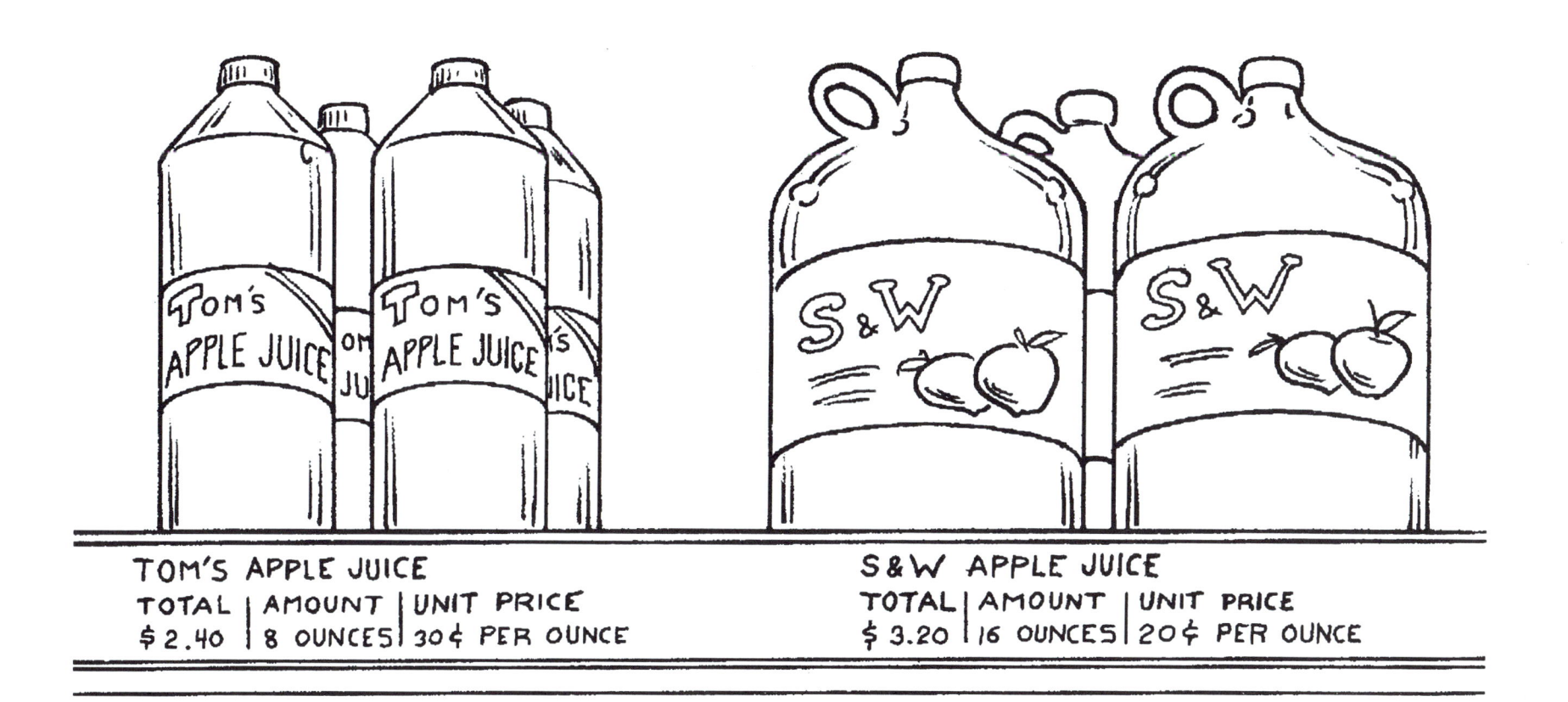

TOM'S APPLE JUICE

TOTAL	AMOUNT	UNIT PRICE
$2.40	8 OUNCES	30¢ PER OUNCE

S&W APPLE JUICE

TOTAL	AMOUNT	UNIT PRICE
$3.20	16 OUNCES	20¢ PER OUNCE

Which costs more money and why?

Read the nutrition label.

Neptune Tuna

Nutrition Facts

Serving Size	1/3 cup
Servings Per Container	3

Amount Per Serving

Calories 80   Calories from Fat 10

	% Daily Value
Total Fat 1g	2%
Saturated Fat 0g	0%
Cholesterol 10g	3%
Sodium 200 mg	8%
Total Carbohydrate 0g	0%
Dietary Fiber 0g	0%
Sugars 0g	
Protein 17g	

Vitamin A 0%	Vitamin C 0%
Calcium 0%	Iron 6%

1. How large is 1 serving?

   _____

2. How many calories are in 1 serving?

   _____

3. How much fat is in 1 serving?

   _____

4. How much protein is in 1 serving?

   _____

5. Is the tuna high in fat?

   _____

6. Is the tuna high in sodium?

   _____

Lesson 6

Save coupons

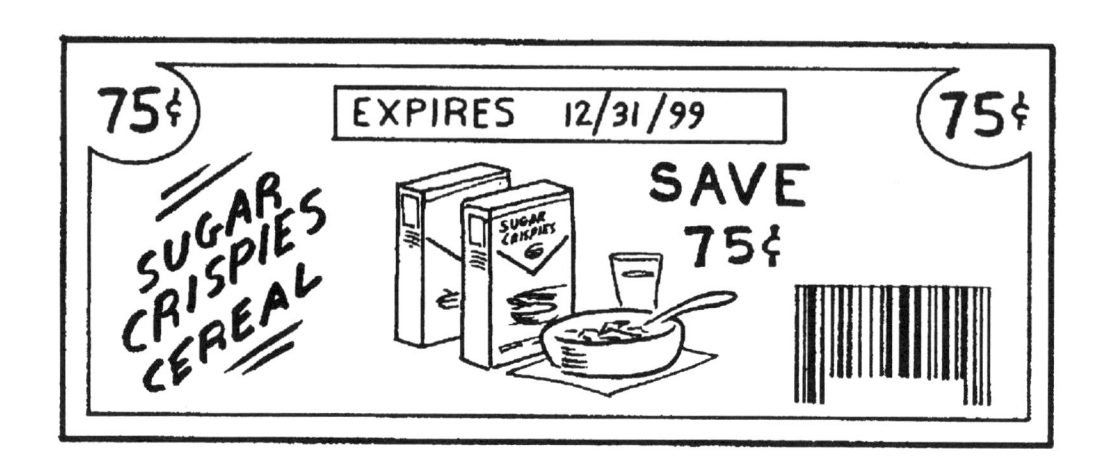

What can you buy with the coupon? _____

What is the expiration date? _____

How much money can you save? _____

Would you use this coupon? _____

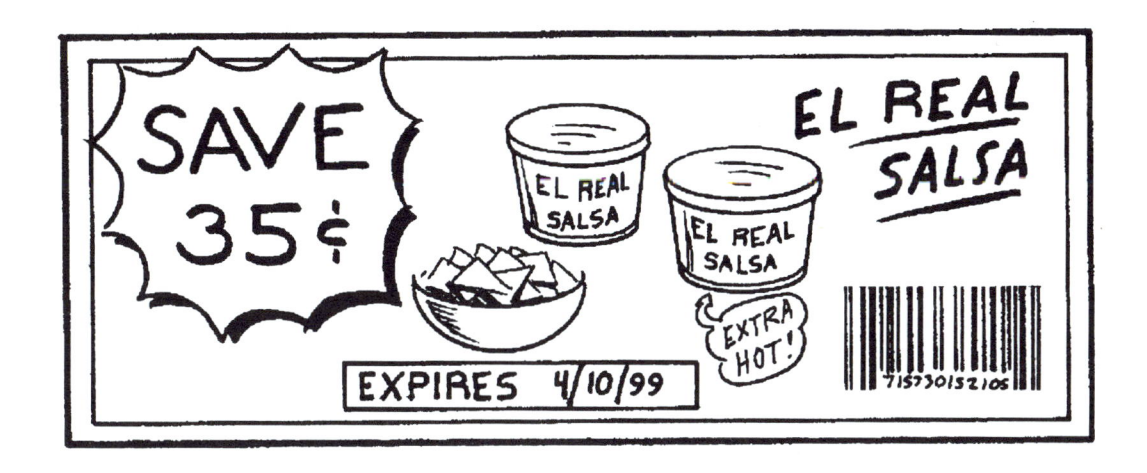

What can you buy with the coupon? _____

What is the expiration date? _____

How much money can you save? _____

Would you use this coupon? _____

Lesson 6

Do coupons always save money?

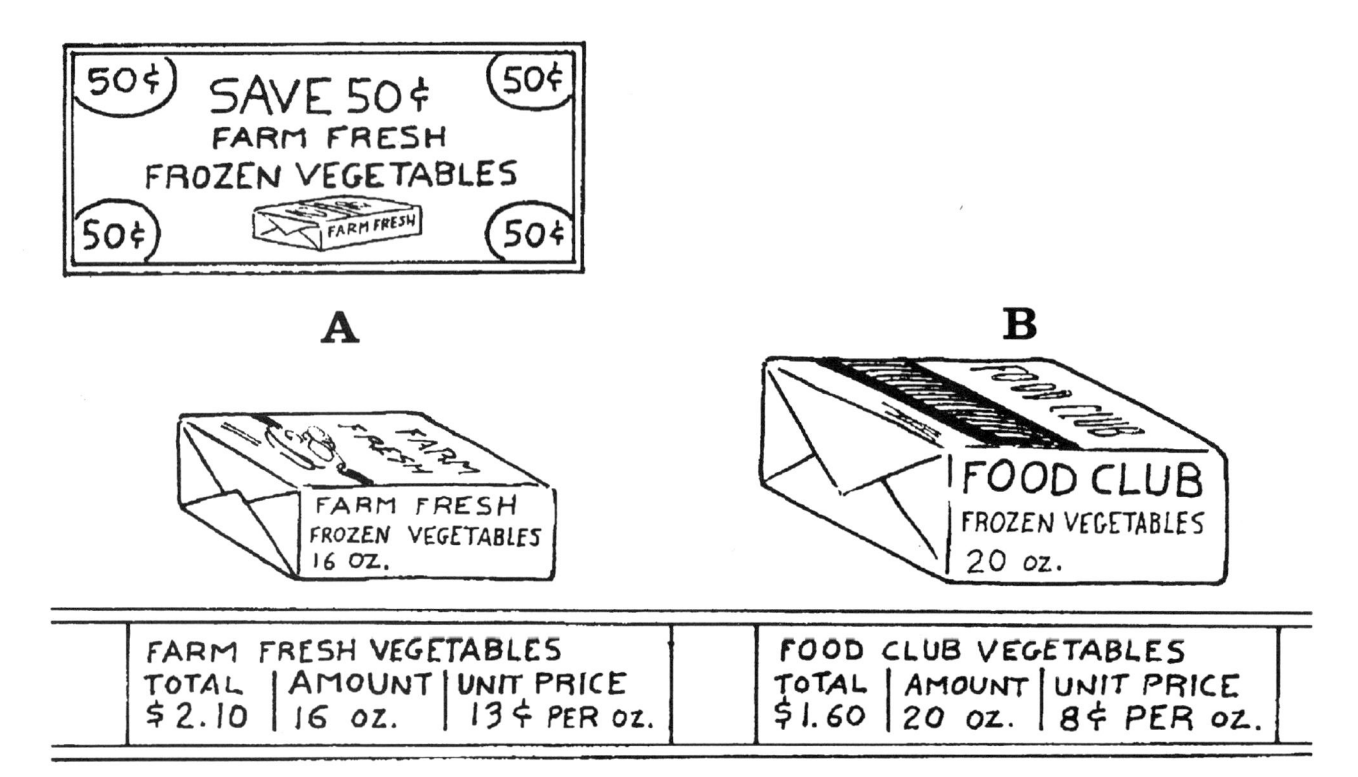

SAVE 50¢ FARM FRESH FROZEN VEGETABLES

A — FARM FRESH FROZEN VEGETABLES 16 OZ.

B — FOOD CLUB FROZEN VEGETABLES 20 oz.

FARM FRESH VEGETABLES		
TOTAL	AMOUNT	UNIT PRICE
$2.10	16 oz.	13¢ PER oz.

FOOD CLUB VEGETABLES		
TOTAL	AMOUNT	UNIT PRICE
$1.60	20 oz.	8¢ PER oz.

1. How much does A cost? _____

2. How much does B cost? _____

3. How much does the coupon save? _____

4. Which costs more money? Why? _____

Advertising

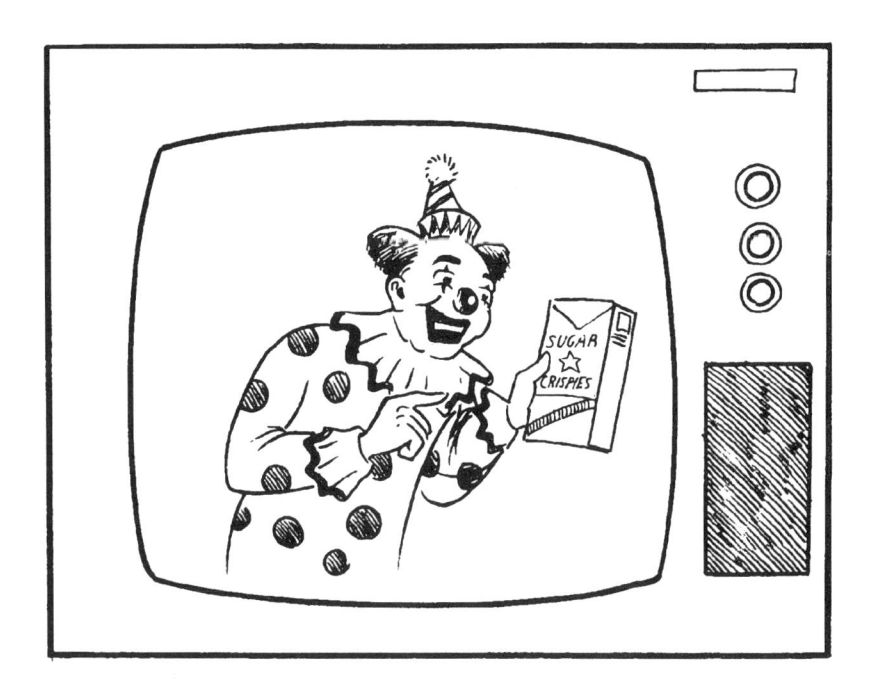

1. What do your children ask you to buy? _____

   _____

2. Do you buy the food you see on television? _____

3. How does television sell food? _____

   _____

Lesson 6

Are you a smart shopper?

Plan ahead. Make a shopping list.

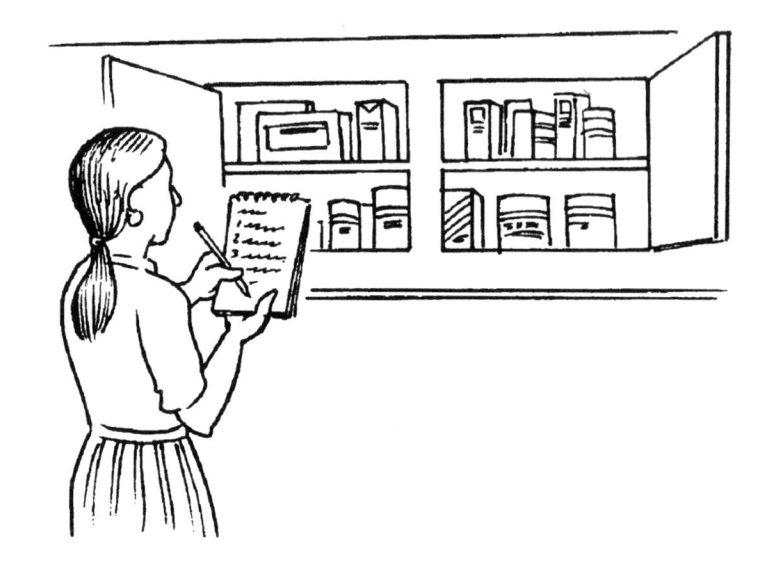

Look at the prices on different brands of food. Store brands cost less.

Look at the prices on different sizes. Larger is often cheaper.

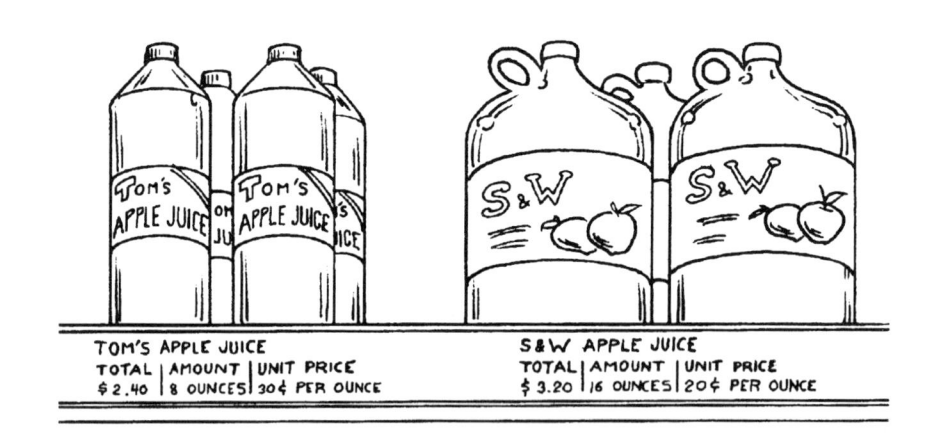

TOM'S APPLE JUICE
TOTAL | AMOUNT | UNIT PRICE
$2.40 | 8 OUNCES | 30¢ PER OUNCE

S&W APPLE JUICE
TOTAL | AMOUNT | UNIT PRICE
$3.20 | 16 OUNCES | 20¢ PER OUNCE

Shop at different stores to look for lower prices.

Look for specials on the foods you buy.

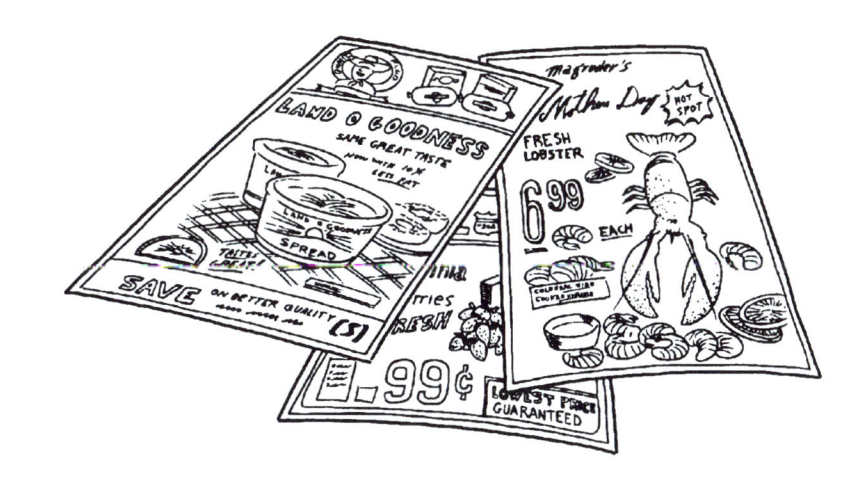

Some package-mixes are more expensive.
They are high in sodium and fat.
Read the label.

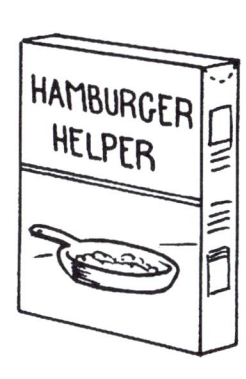

Food costs more at a convenience store.

Food	Supermarket	Convenience Store
milk	$0.46 a quart	$0.85 a quart
bread	$1.15 a loaf	$1.35 a loaf

Lesson 6

Joan is giving a dinner party.

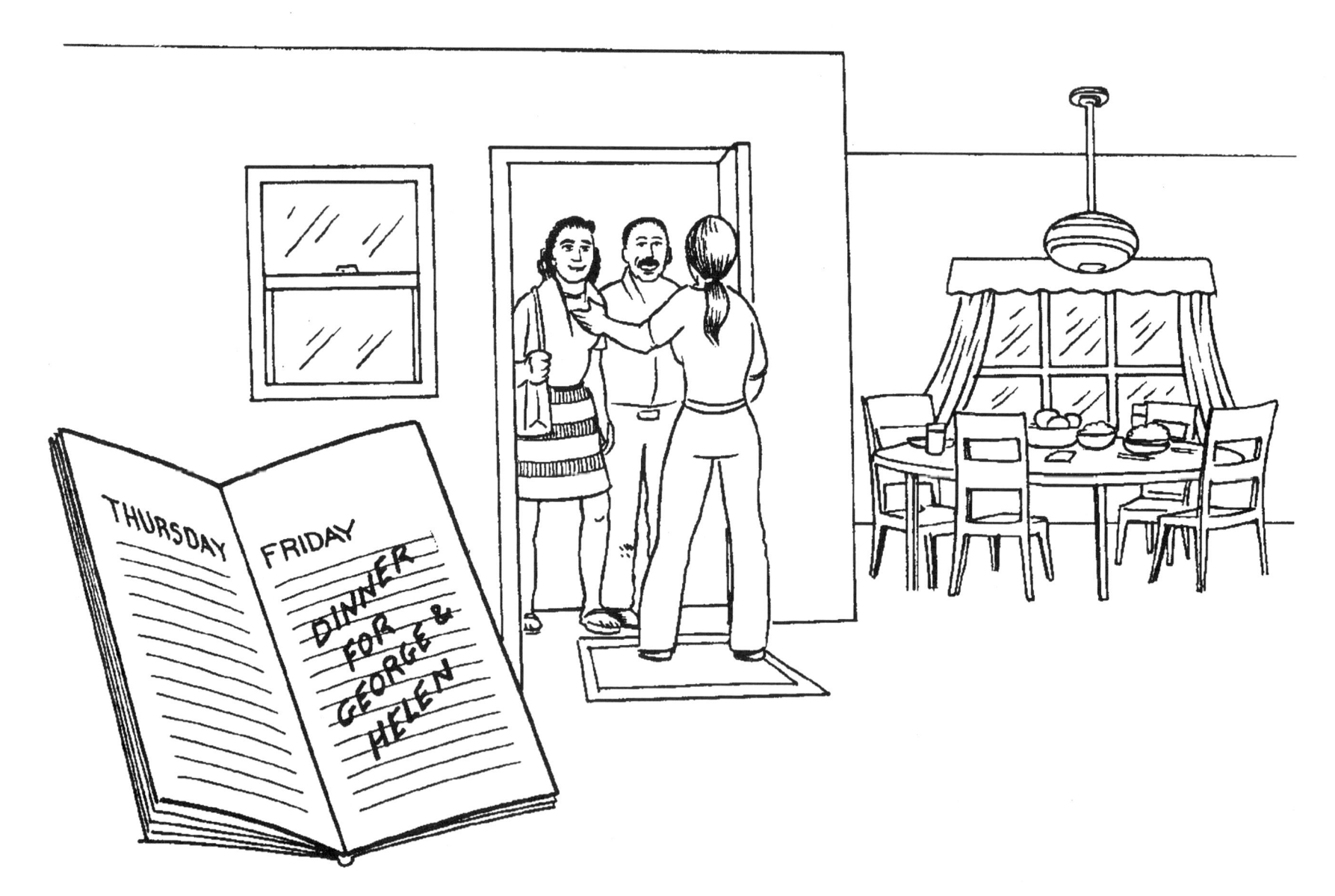

Lesson 6

Help Joan plan a menu. Next, make a shopping list for her. Use newspaper ads for specials, coupons, the food pyramid, and the shopping tips on pages 90-91.

Menu

Things to buy...

Is your dinner low in fat?

Is it high in fiber?

Is it low in sodium?

Lesson 6

A Healthy Recipe

Macaroni Salad

2 cups cooked macaroni
1/4 cup sliced celery
1/4 cup chopped carrot
2 tablespoons chopped onion

1 tablespoon mayonnaise
1 teaspoon vinegar
1 teaspoon mustard
1/8 teaspoon pepper

1. Cook macaroni.

2. Slice celery.

3. Chop carrot and onion.

4. Mix macaroni, celery, carrot, and onion in a large bowl.

5. Mix mayonnaise, vinegar, mustard, and pepper in a small bowl. *Makes 4 servings.*

1 2 3 4 5 6 **7** 8

Eat Well and Stay Healthy

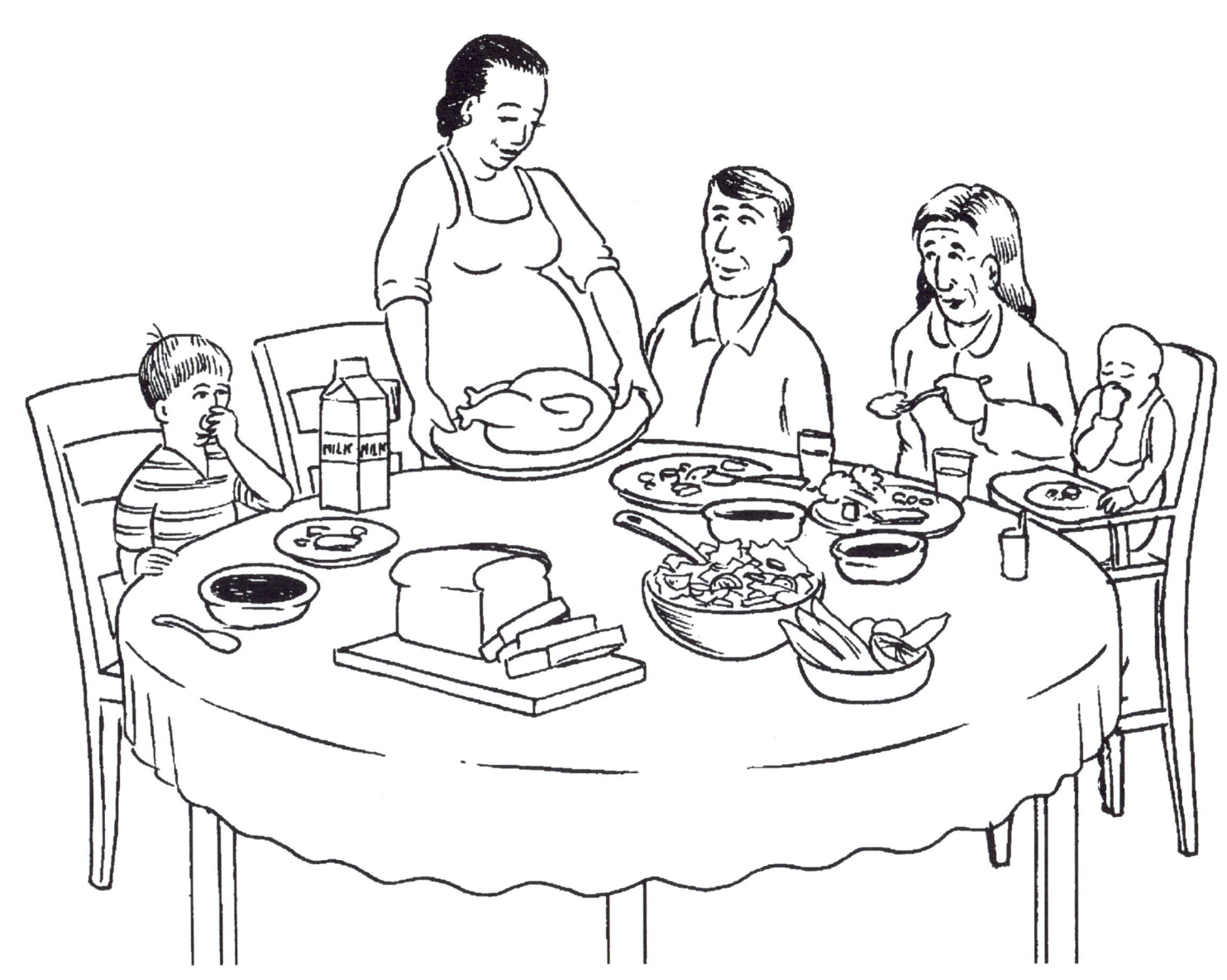

Do you eat well?

Make a check under your answer.

	always	sometimes	never
1. Do you eat foods from each food group?			
2. Do you watch your weight?			
3. Do you eat lowfat foods?			
4. Do you drink water?			
5. Do you use caffeine?			
6. Do you eat foods with fiber?			
7. Do you drink alcohol?			
8. Do you exercise?			
9. Do you smoke?			
10. Do you use salt?			

Eating well can help us stay healthy.

Doctors don't know why we get some diseases.

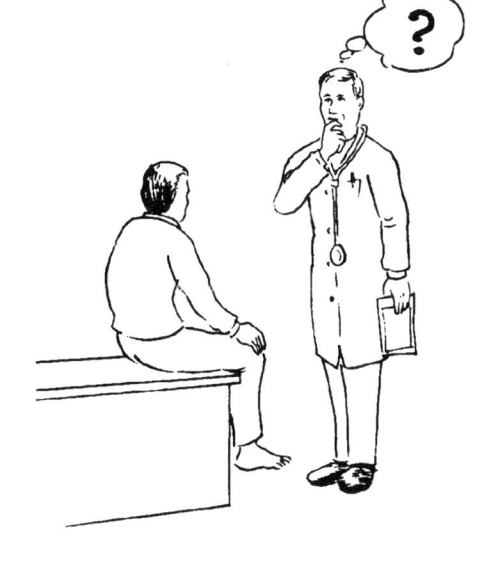

But, doctor's say . . . .

There are some diseases we may get from eating a bad diet. Those diseases are

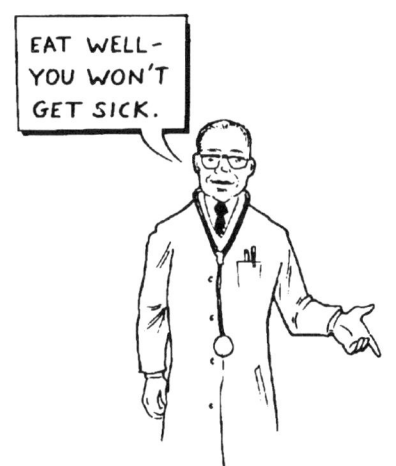

    high blood pressure

    heart disease

    diabetes

    cancer

High Blood Pressure

High blood pressure makes it hard for blood to go through the veins and arteries.

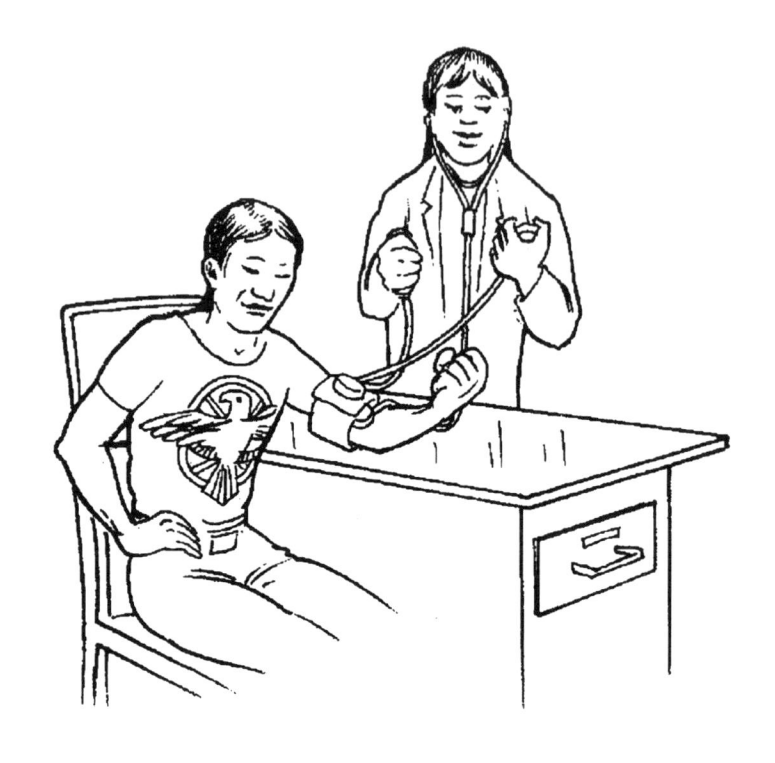

Eat less salt and sodium. Most people need only ¼ teaspoon (500 milligrams) of sodium each day. Don't use salt at the table.

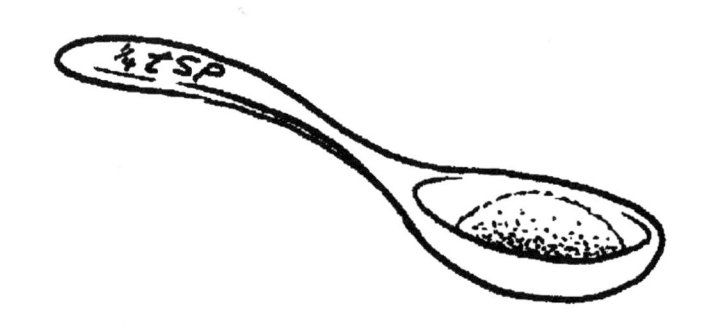

Lesson 7

These foods are high in salt.

Food	Sodium per serving (mg)
chicken dinner (fast food)	2,243
tomato sauce	1,498
canned chili con carne	1,194
soy sauce	1,029

These foods are also high in sodium.

canned foods	ham	garlic salt
pickles	sausage	onion salt
dried meat or fish	potato chips	MSG
adobo		

Eat small amounts of salty snacks.

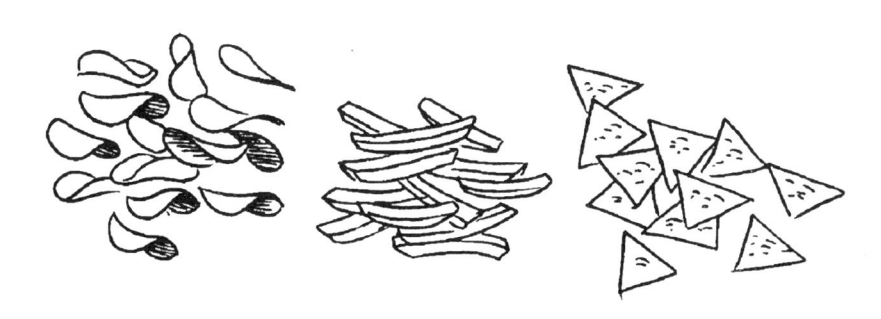

Heart Disease

Heart disease means your heart has to work too hard to pump blood.

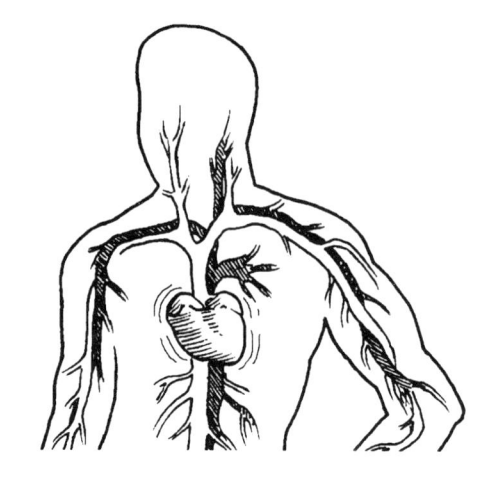

Eat less fat, salt, and sugar.

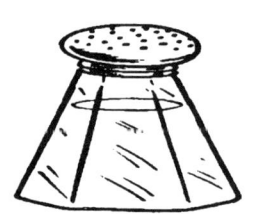

Exercise three times a week for 20 minutes.

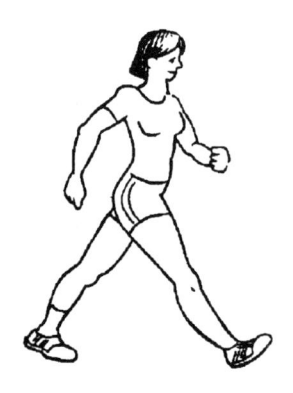

Lesson 7

Watch your weight.

Don't smoke.

Take time to rest.

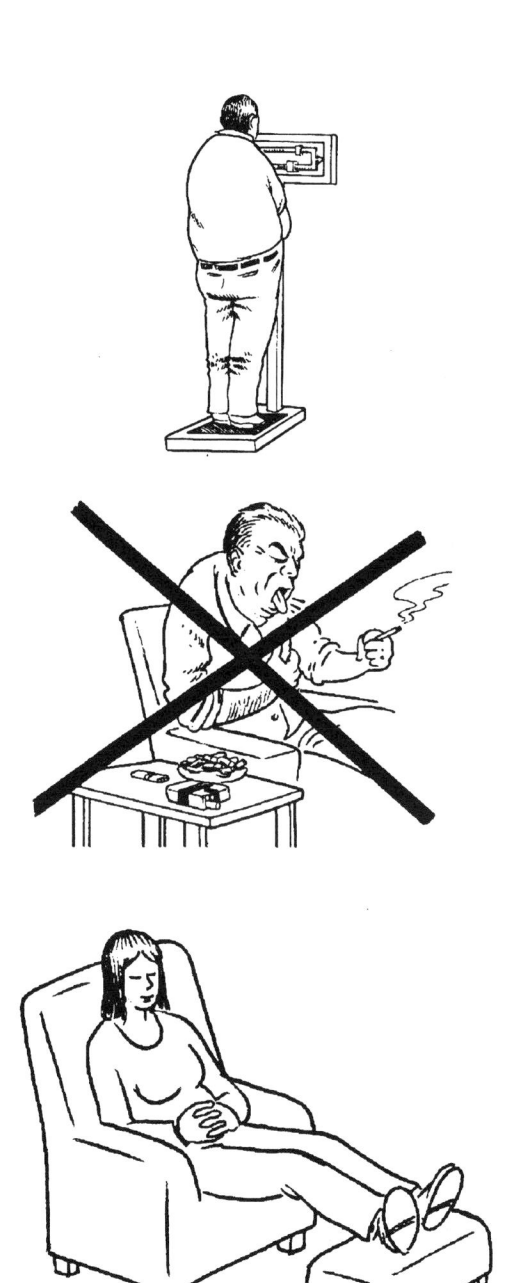

Diabetes

Diabetes means there is too much sugar in the blood.

Eat regular meals.

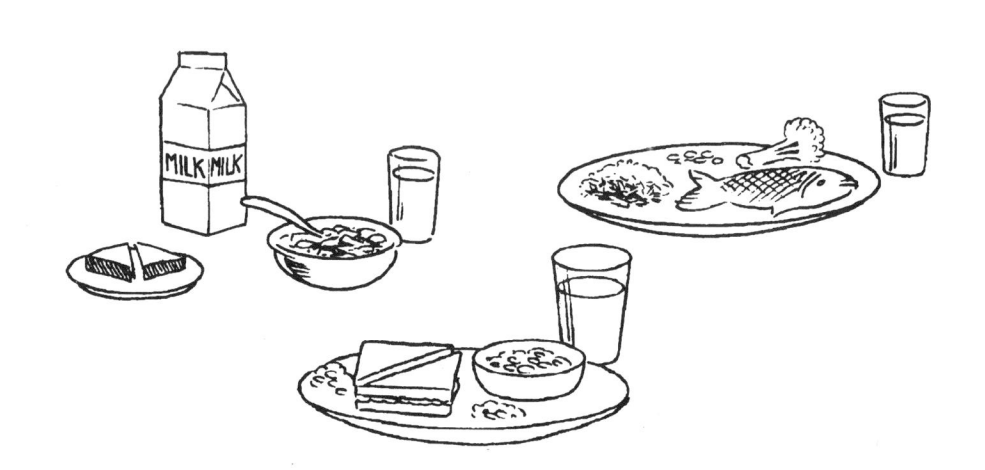

Eat less sugar.

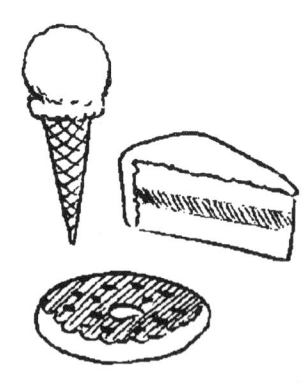

Lesson 7

Eat less fat.

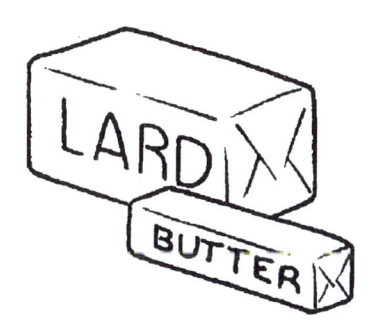

Eat more fiber.

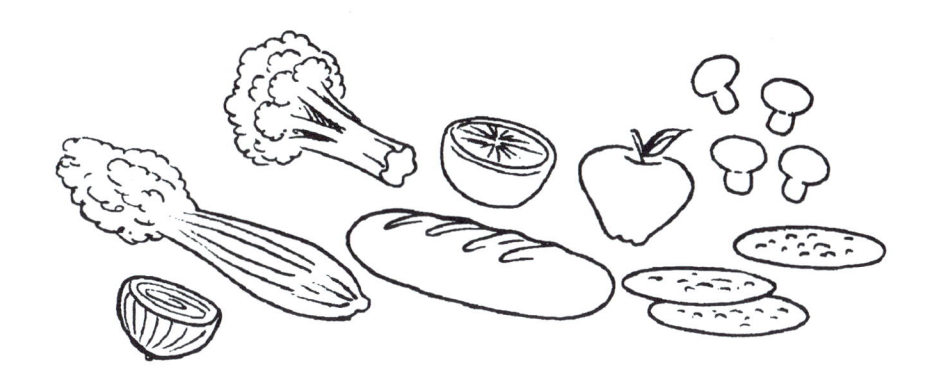

Watch your weight.

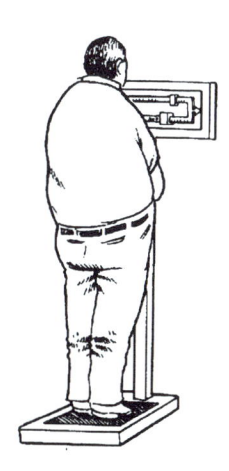

Cancer

Cancer makes cells grow too quickly. This stops the body from working.

Eat less fat.

Use small amounts of fatty foods.

Eat high-fiber foods.

Eat fruits and vegetables with the skin.

Eat foods with vitamins A and C.

Vitamin A — dark green vegetables, deep yellow fruits and vegetables.

Vitamin C — citrus fruits, strawberries, melons, broccoli, cauliflower, and green peppers.

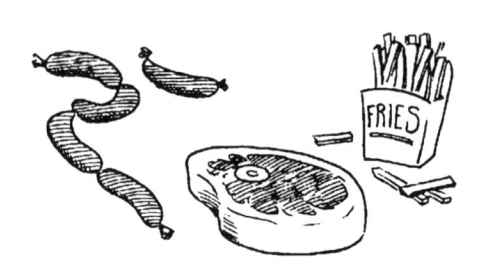

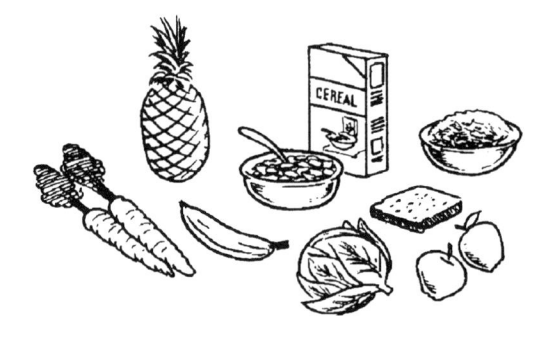

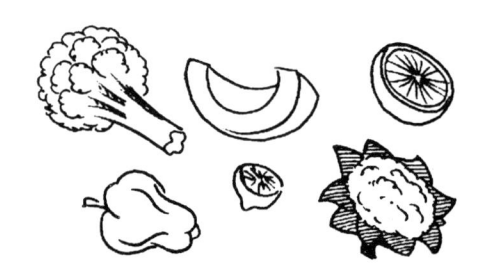

Eat vegetables from the cabbage family.

the cabbage family = bok choy, brussel sprouts, turnips, broccoli, cabbage

Drink less alcohol.

Eat fewer salt-cured, smoked, and nitrite-cured foods.

Watch your weight.

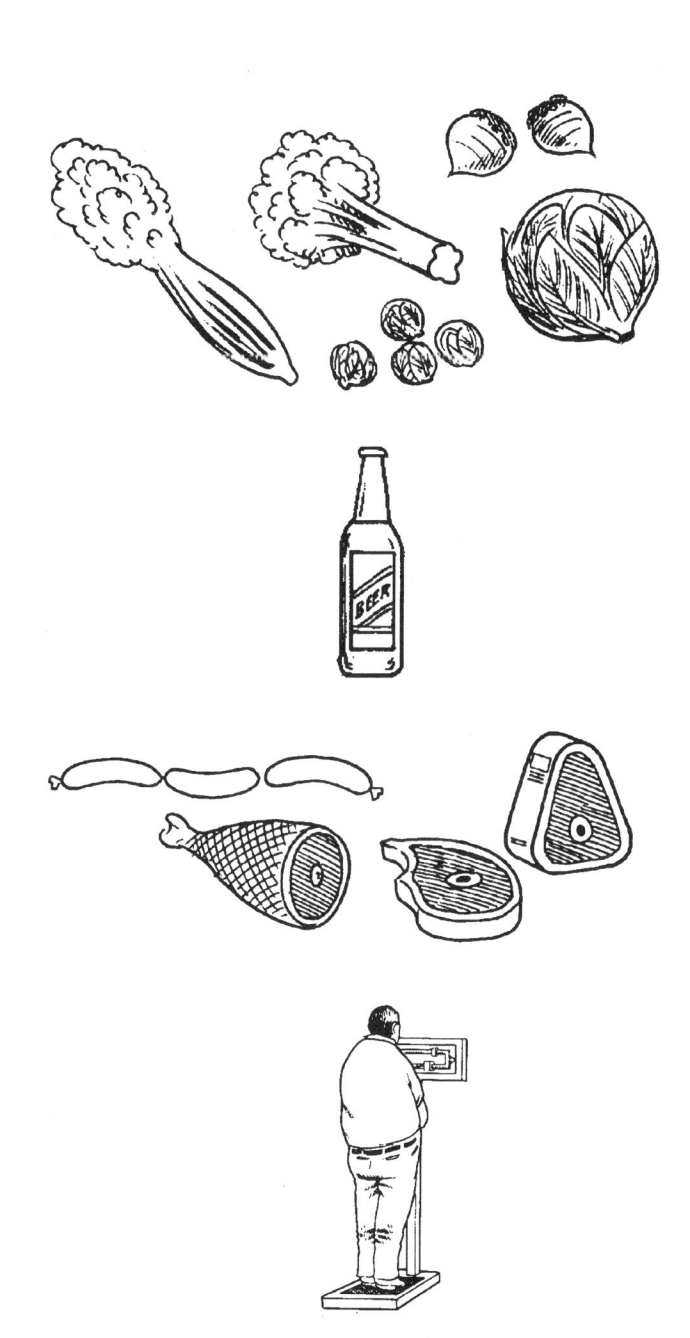

Lesson 7

Fruit with Yogurt Dip

8 ounces vanilla non-fat yogurt

8 ounces strawberry non-fat yogurt

cinnamon

1 banana

1 pint of strawberries

2 apples

1. Mix vanilla yogurt with strawberry yogurt in a bowl.

2. Sprinkle the yogurt with cinnamon.

3. Slice the banana lengthwise and in half.

4. Remove the stems from the strawberries.

5. Cut the apples into wedges.

6. Place the fruit around the bowl of yogurt.

7. Dip the fruit into the yogurt and eat. *Makes 4 servings.*

1 2 3 4 5 6 7 **8**

Get the Help You Need

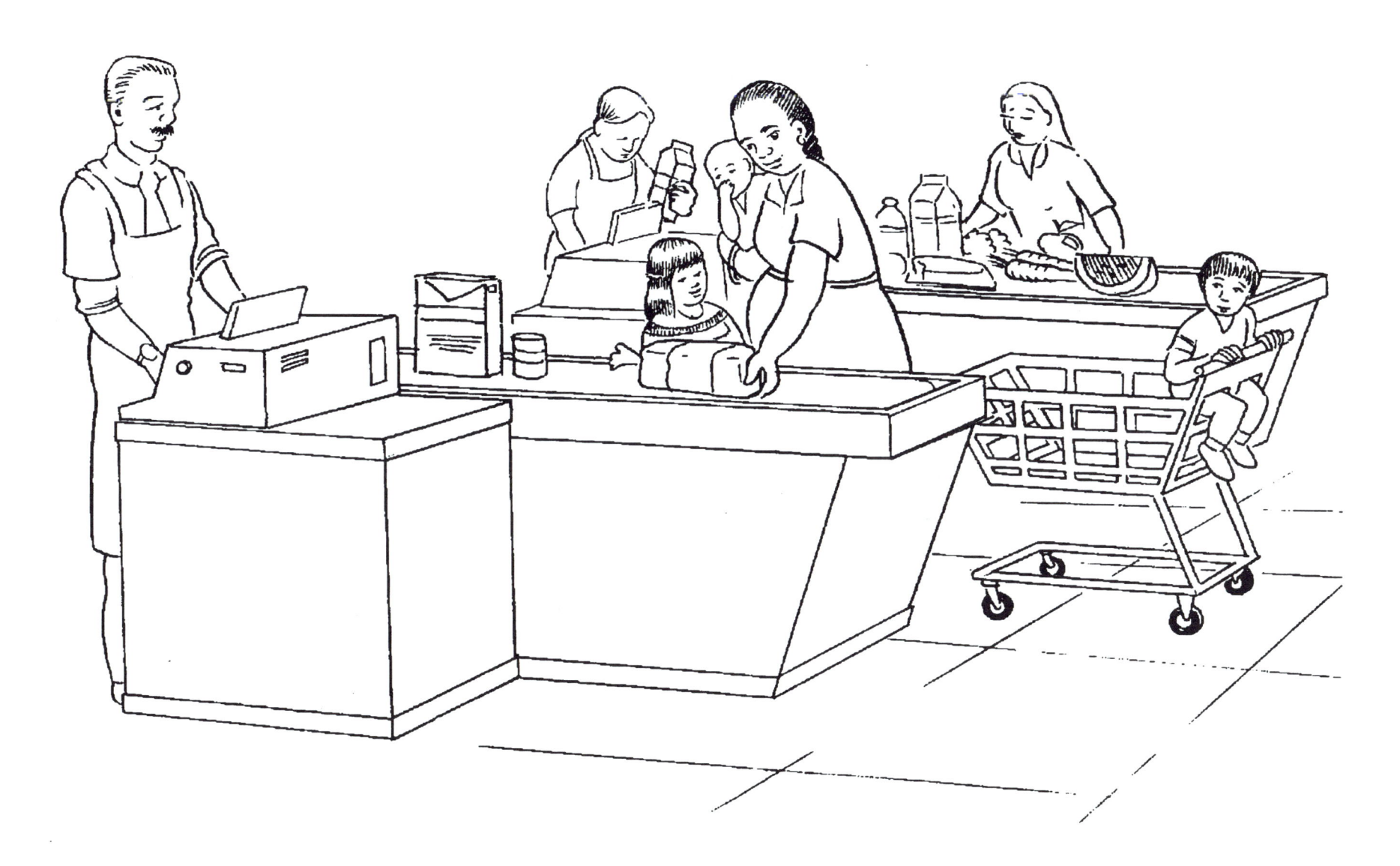

Lesson 8

Pregnant women must eat well.

Pregnant women should

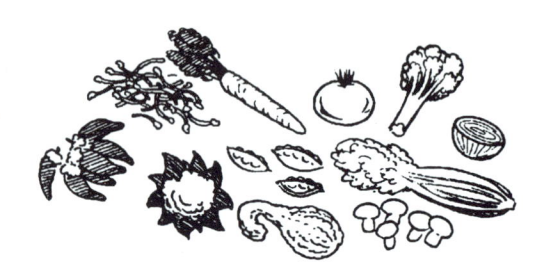

eat more fruits and vegetables

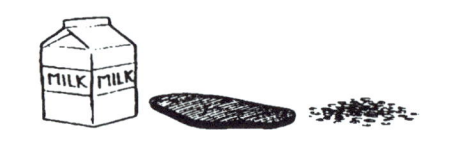

eat more foods with iron and calcium

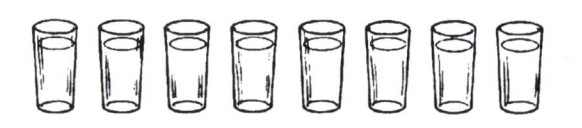

drink 8-10 glasses of fluid a day

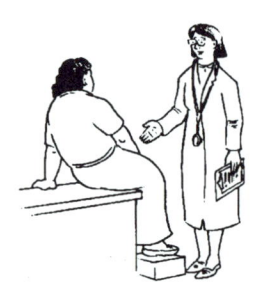

see your doctor.

For a Healthy Baby

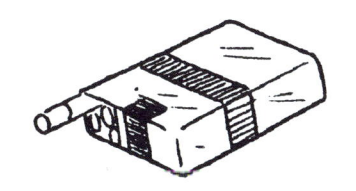

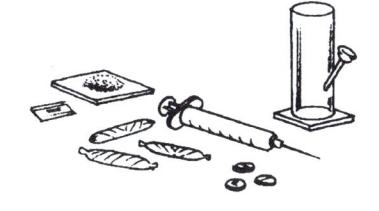

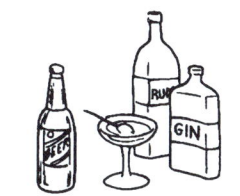

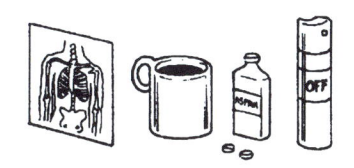

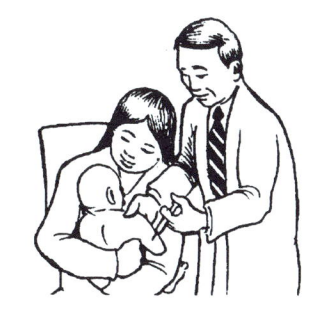

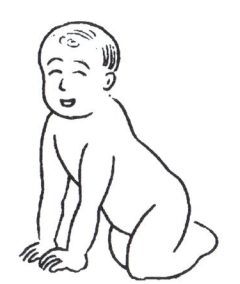

Don't smoke.

Don't drink alcohol.

Don't take drugs.

Ask the doctor about medicine, chemicals caffeine, and x-rays.

And remember to immunize your baby.

Lesson 8

Feeding your Baby

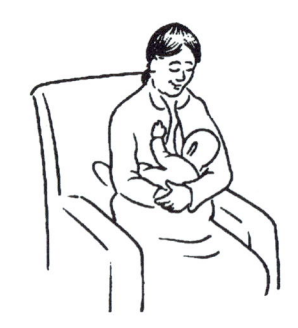

0-6 months — Breastfeed, if possible. Do not give your baby solid foods.

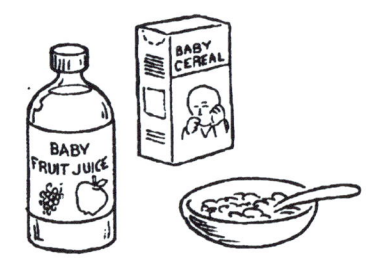

6-7 months — Give your baby cereals, mashed fruits and juices.

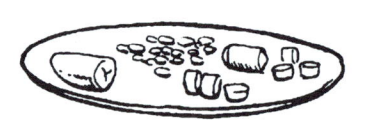

8-12 months — Add meats, yogurt, and egg yolks. Cut food in small pieces for your baby to eat.

after 12 months — You can now feed your child the foods you eat.

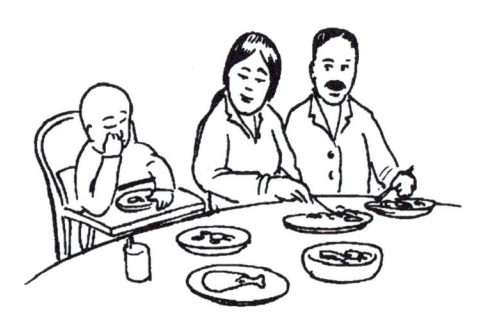

Feeding Your Child

Your child needs foods from each of the food groups.

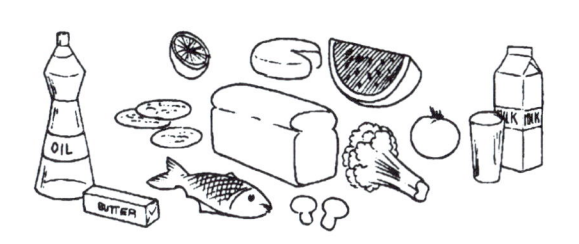

Give your child small servings. Offer second servings.

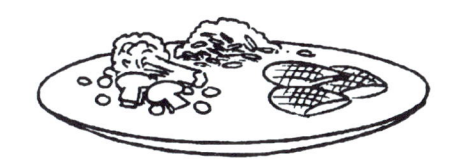

Your child may get hungry. Snacks are important.

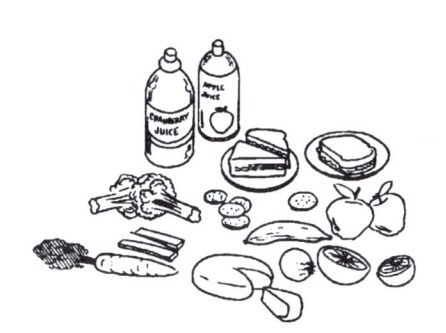

These foods can be bad for your child's teeth.

    soda   chocolate

    potato chips   pies, cakes, cookies

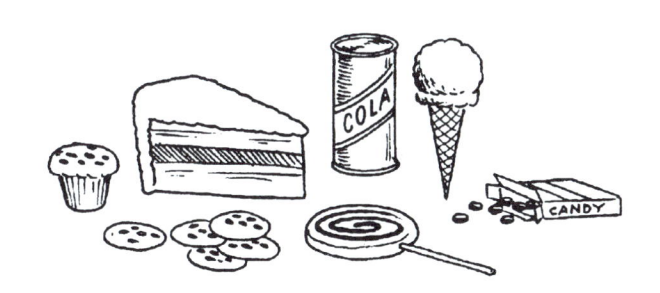

    candy   gum

Can you get help from WIC?

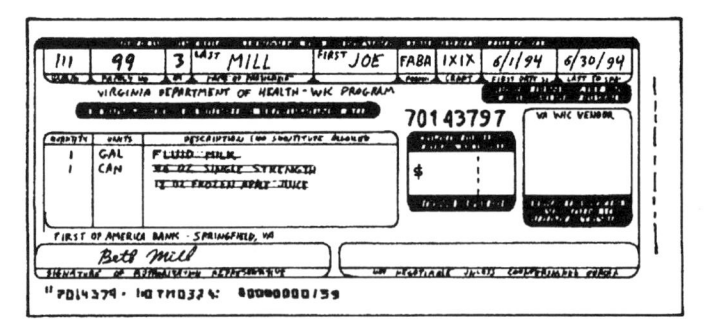

**Women, Infants, and Children (WIC) is a government program.
WIC can help you buy food.**

Circle your answers.

1. Are you a pregnant or breastfeeding woman?   Yes   No

2. Do you have a child under 5 years old?   Yes   No

3. Do you need money for food?   Yes   No

4. Do you have health problems?   Yes   No
   or
   Does your child have health problems?   Yes   No

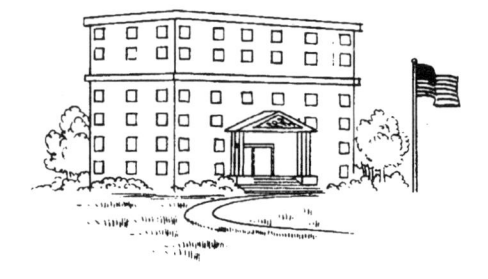

Go to the WIC office for an application and an interview.

WIC gives

health classes

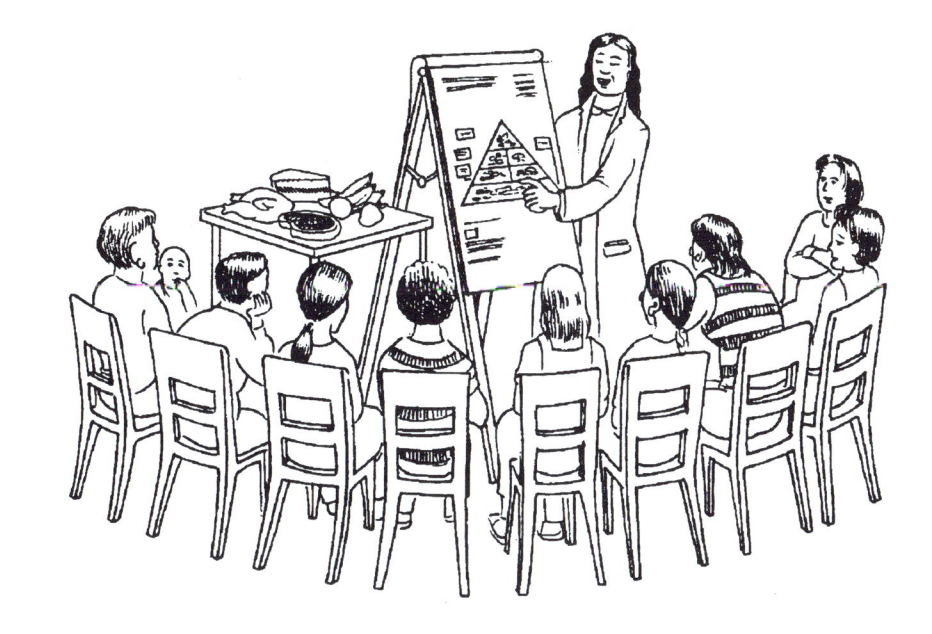

health services

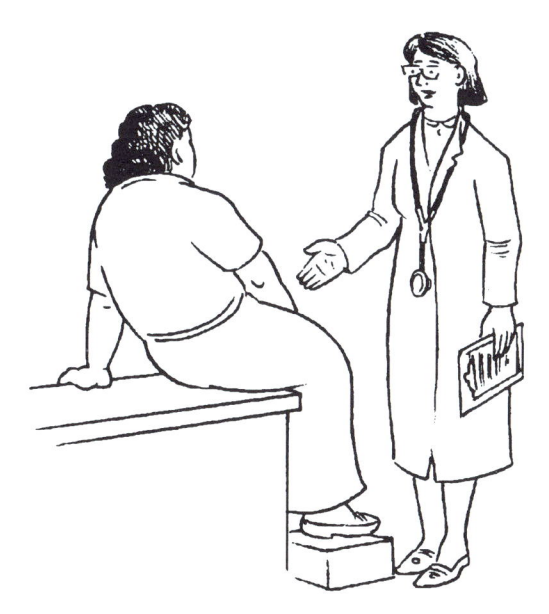

Lesson 8

WIC checks can buy

baby cereal

baby fruit juice

baby formula

beans

carrots

cheese

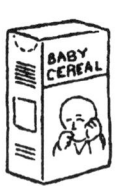

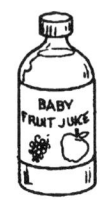

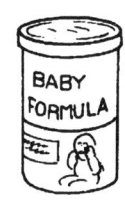

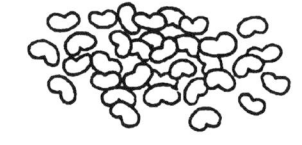

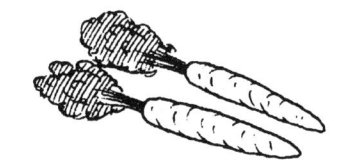

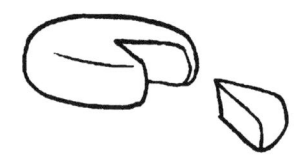

Lesson 8

eggs

fruit juice

milk

cereal

peanut butter

tuna

U.S. Government Food Stamps can help you buy food.

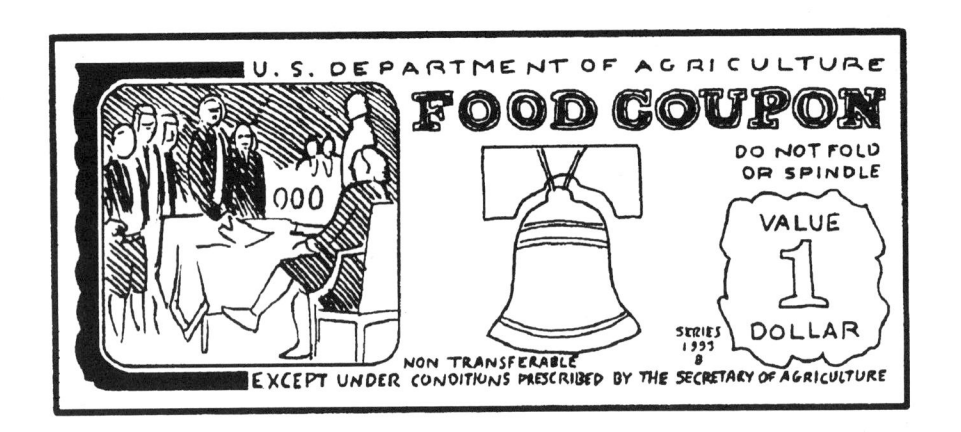

Food Stamps can buy

food

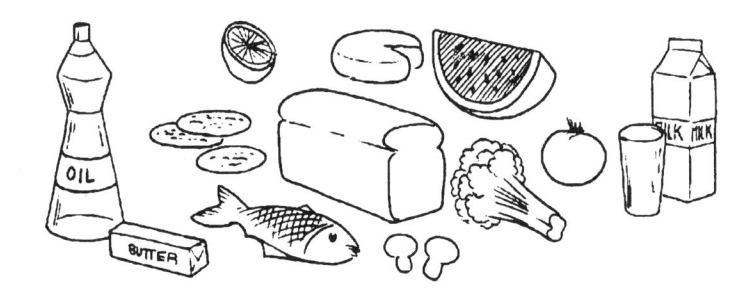

seeds and plants that grow food

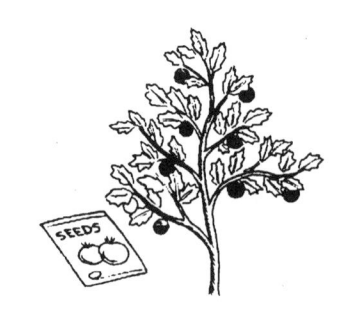

Food Stamps can't buy

alcohol

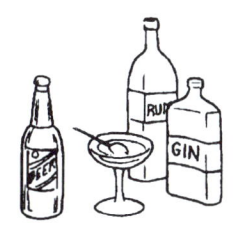

cigarettes

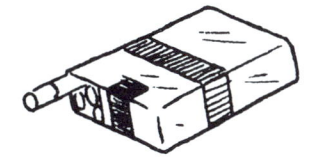

vitamins and minerals

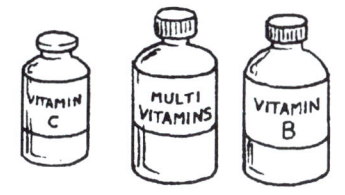

dog and cat food

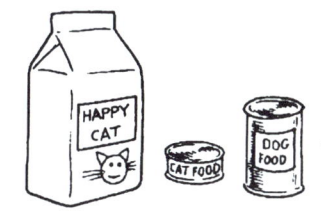

soap and paper things

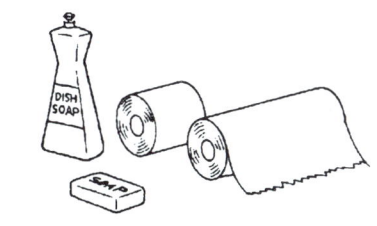

Can Sung get Food Stamps?

Sung does not have a job. He has no money for food. He gets welfare. Sung has a green card.

He does not have a home. Can Sung get Food Stamps?

Food Stamps is a government program. You can get Food Stamps if you..

     1. are a U.S. citizen or have a green card

     2. have no money for food

     3. are on welfare

     4. are homeless

Sung must go to the Food Stamp Office for an application and an interview.

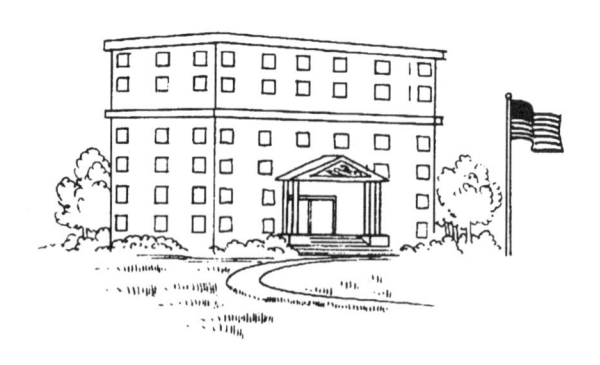

Churches and Community Groups

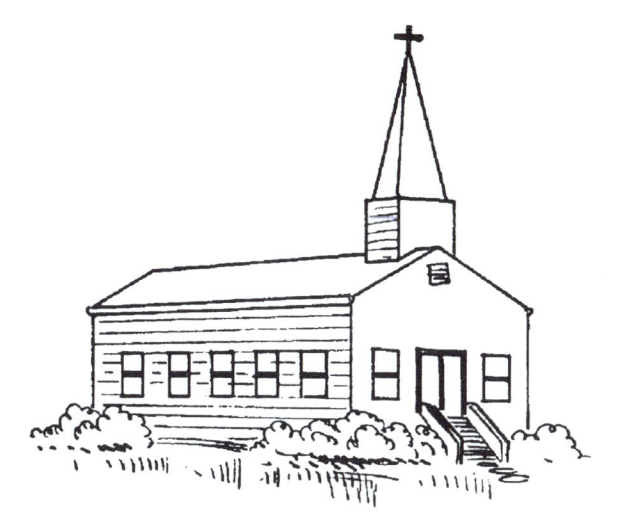

Churches can help you get food.

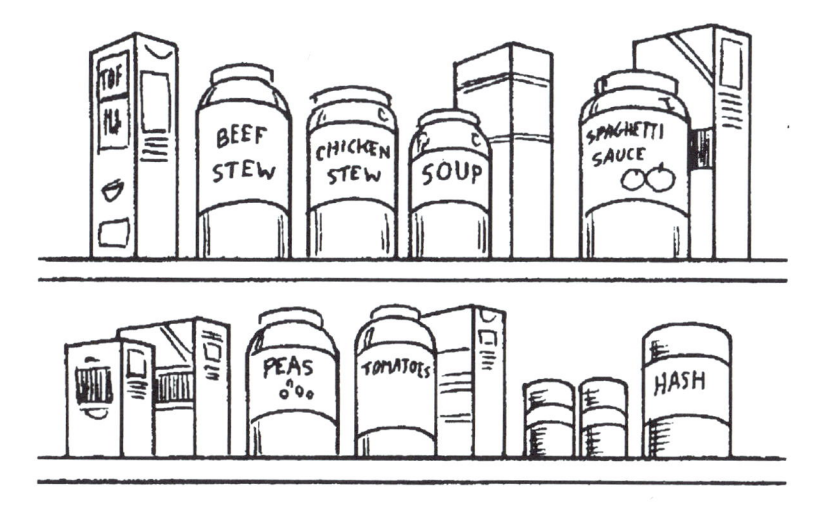

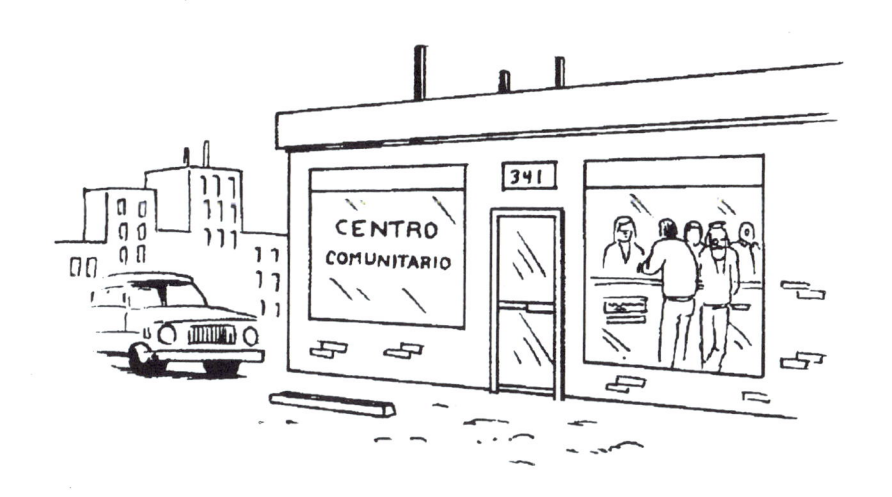

Community groups can help you get food.

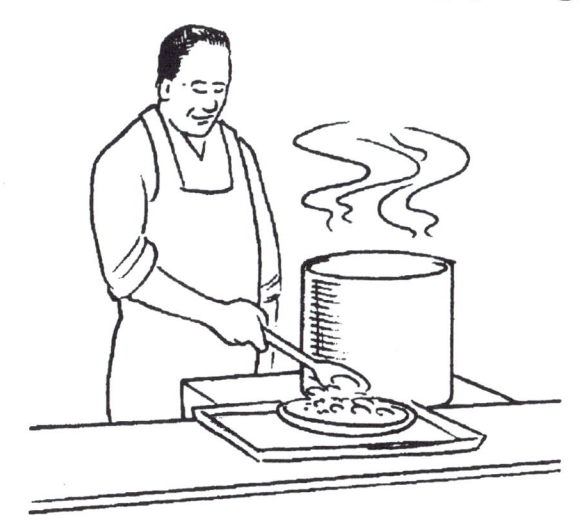

They have food banks.

They have soup kitchens.

Lesson 8

Telephone Numbers

WIC Office: _____

Food Stamp Office: _____

Community Health Center: _____

Food Bank or Soup Kitchen: _____

Farmworker Organization: _____

Police Station: _____

Poison Control Center: _____

Other: _____

_____

_____

Write your own recipe.

Lesson 8

Your Word List

GLOSSARY OF FOODS

Food	Serving	fat(g)	calories	fiber(g)	sodium(mg)
apple					
whole	1 medium	0.4	81	4	1
juice	1 cup	0.3	116	1	7
applesauce	1/2 cup	0.1	53	2	0
avocado	1 (6 oz.)	30	306	4	21
banana	1 medium	0.6	105	2	1
beans (legumes)					
all types, cooked	1/2 cup	0.4	124	1	9
beer	12 oz	0	148	0	19
Big Mac (McDonalds)	1	26	500	1	890
bread (multigrain)	1 slice	0.9	70	2	103
bean burrito (Taco Bell)	1	14	381	1	1148
cake					
chocolate, with frosting	1 piece	17.0	388	2	648
white, with frosting	1 piece	14.6	369	1	420
pound	1 piece	9.0	200	1	110
angel	1 piece	0.2	161	0	161

Glossary of Foods

Food	Serving	fat(g)	calories	fiber(g)	sodium(mg)
cheese (cheddar)	1 oz.	9.4	114	0	176
chicken					
with skin, fried	1/2 breast	10.7	236	0	77
w/o skin, roasted	1/2 breast	3.1	142	0	70
leg, fried	1 leg	8.7	120	0	92
chocolate bar (snickers)	1 oz.	6.5	135	1	75
coffee	8 oz.	0	4	0	4
carbonated sodas	12 oz.	0	152	0	14
sugar free	12 oz.	0	1	0	8
corn					
corn on the cob	1 medium	0.9	83	4	4
cooked	1/2 cup	1.1	89	5	14
frozen, cooked	1/2 cup	0.2	67	4	4
cream style, canned	1/2 cup	0.4	93	4	365
egg fried w/ 1tsp. fat	1 large	7.8	104	0	144
fish (haddock)					
cooked	3 1/2 oz.	0.6	79	0	58
fried	3 1/2 oz.	10.0	180	0	130
smoked/canned	3 1/2 oz.	0.4	103	0	655
french fries (McDonalds)	1 order, large	21.6	400	1	200

Glossary of Foods

Food	Serving	fat(g)	calories	fiber(g)	sodium(mg)
ice cream					
chocolate	1/2 cup	7.2	134	1	58
strawberry	1/2 cup	6.0	128	0	55
lamb					
leg, lean	3 1/2 oz.	8.1	180	0	60
lean & marbled	3 1/2 oz.	14.5	242	0	52
macaroni (semolina)	1 cup	0.7	159	1	1
milk					
whole	1 cup	8.0	150	0	122
lowfat (2%)	1 cup	4.7	121	0	123
skim	1 cup	0.4	86	0	126
noodles					
egg	1 cup	2.4	200	1	3
ramen	1 cup	6.5	188	1	978
rice	1 cup	0	140	1	0
spaghetti	1 cup	1.0	159	1	1
pizza-cheese (Dominos)	2 slices	10	360	NA	1000
plantain, cooked	1 cup	0.3	179	1	8
pork					
loin chop, lean	1 chop	7.7	170	0	40
loin chop, lean & fat	1 chop	22.5	314	0	63

Glossary of Foods

Food	Serving	fat(g)	calories	fiber(g)	sodium(mg)
potato chips	1 oz.-14 chips	11.2	159	1	182
rice					
white	1/2 cup	1.2	111	0	0
fried	1/2	7.2	181	1	550
strawberries	1 cup	0.2	45	3	2
tomato					
raw	1 medium	0.3	24	1	10
stewed	1/2 cup	0.2	34	1	325
paste, canned	1/2 cup	1.2	110	4	86
tortilla					
(corn, not fried)	1 medium	0.8	48	1	38
flour	1 medium	2.5	59	1	63
tortilla chips	1 oz-10 chips	6.6	139	0	140
whiskey	1 fl. oz.	0	70	0	0
wine	4 fl. oz.	0	85	0	0
yogurt					
lowfat, vanilla	1 cup	2.8	194	0	149
nonfat, plain	1 cup	0.4	127	0	174